SEX *in the* WORLD *of* MYTH

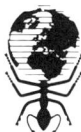

SEX
in the
WORLD
of
MYTH

DAVID LEEMING

REAKTION BOOKS

For Pam

Published by

REAKTION BOOKS LTD
Unit 32, Waterside
44–48 Wharf Road
London N1 7UX, UK
www.reaktionbooks.co.uk

First published 2018
Copyright © David Leeming 2018

Printed and bound in China by 1010 Printing International Ltd

A catalogue record for this book is available from the British Library

ISBN 978 1 78023 977 4

Contents

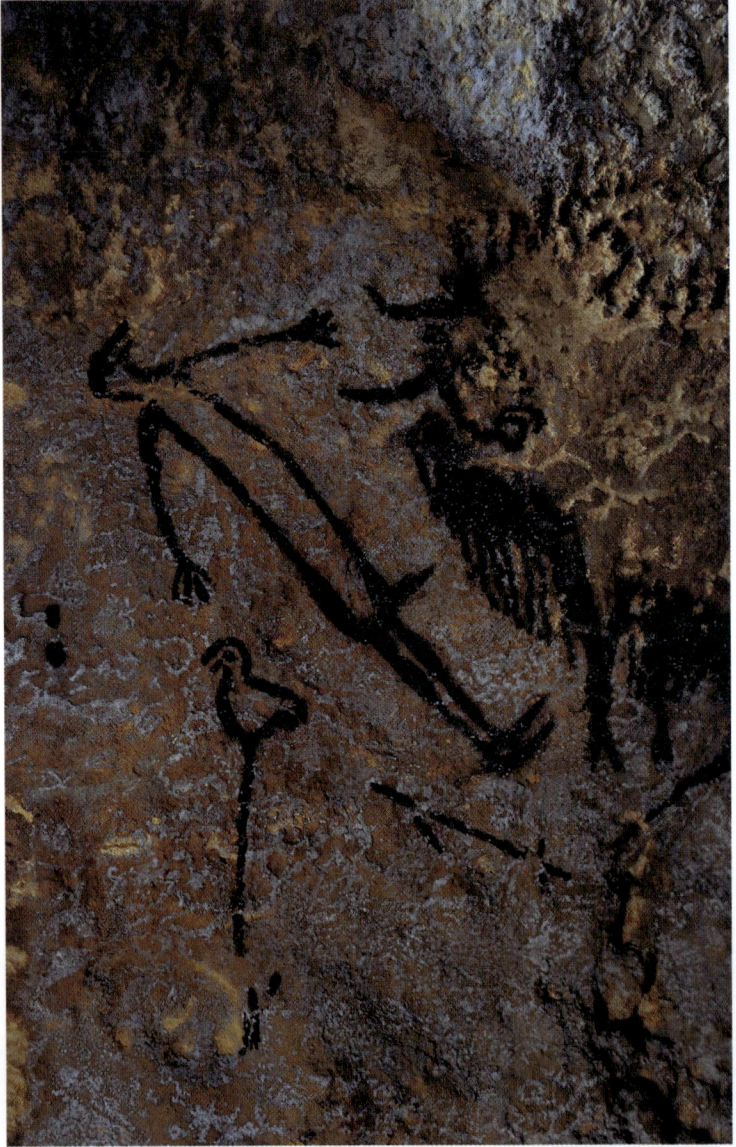

The Shaft Scene, Lascaux Cave painting, *c.* 17,000 BCE.

Preface

THE APPROACH TO the subject of sex in myth will naturally involve explorations of mythologies from many sections of the world. This does not mean that all mythologies give equal time to sexual matters. Mythologies reflect our various individual and cultural approaches to sex. Like individuals, there are mythologies which revel in sexual stories, and others that are distinctly modest or even prudish where sex is concerned. I have not been able, of course, to include every culture or civilization, but I have covered the mythologies of several great civilizations of the past as well as lesser-known cultures in which sex plays a significant role. I have begun with the seminal civilizations of the Middle East and have moved from there to the Indo-European cultures of Europe and India, followed by the primarily animistic traditions of Asia, Africa, Oceania and the Americas.

The reader should not be surprised to find the myths of Christians, Jews and Hindus placed in the company of those of the ancient Greeks and Egyptians and those of such cultures as the African Dogon and the Native American Navajo. Sex is sex everywhere. All humans, and therefore all cultures, are concerned with it. Some tell explicit stories about it, while some veil these stories in metaphor. Some myths celebrate sex as the very reason for existence;

some clearly despair of its power over our lives; some consider it inherently evil and demeaning; some find complex paths to denying it altogether.

The mythologies to which I have given most space are those that have been expressed fully in the written word. The characteristics and activities of the deities and heroes of Mesopotamia, Egypt, Israel, Canaan, Greece, Rome and India are revealed in detail in elaborate texts such as the Sumerian hymns to Inanna, the Babylonian *Enuma Elish*, the *Epic of Gilgamesh*, the Bible, the works of Homer, Hesiod, Aeschylus, Sophocles and Ovid, and the Vedas and epics of India. As it happens, these are the mythologies most concerned with sex.

The mythologies treated in much shorter chapters are generally those of animistic traditions in which deities and their activities are less clearly defined – mythologies such as those of sub-Saharan Africa, Oceania and the Americas, and even China and Japan, which have been given some literary exposure only long after the establishment of the myths themselves. We have a much more intimate knowledge of Inanna, Gilgamesh, Medusa and Shiva than, for instance, of the Japanese goddess Amaterasu, the African trickster Ananse or the Native American Kokopelli, because of the strong literary traditions that have exposed them to us. In treating the mythologies of Africa, the Americas and, to some extent, Oceania, we are faced with such a large number of individual tribal groups that it has been necessary to consider these groups collectively, taking examples of sexual myths from large geographic areas.

As I have explored the sexual myths I have suggested ways in which these myths reveal cultural priorities, particularly in connection with gender relations and gender identity. In short, I have considered ways in which sex in myths has been used metaphorically for theological or moral purposes, or to justify cultural traditions. The tendency to compare as we move from one culture to another, however, leads inevitably to a consideration in a concluding chapter of certain universal themes that suggest a generally human myth of sex.

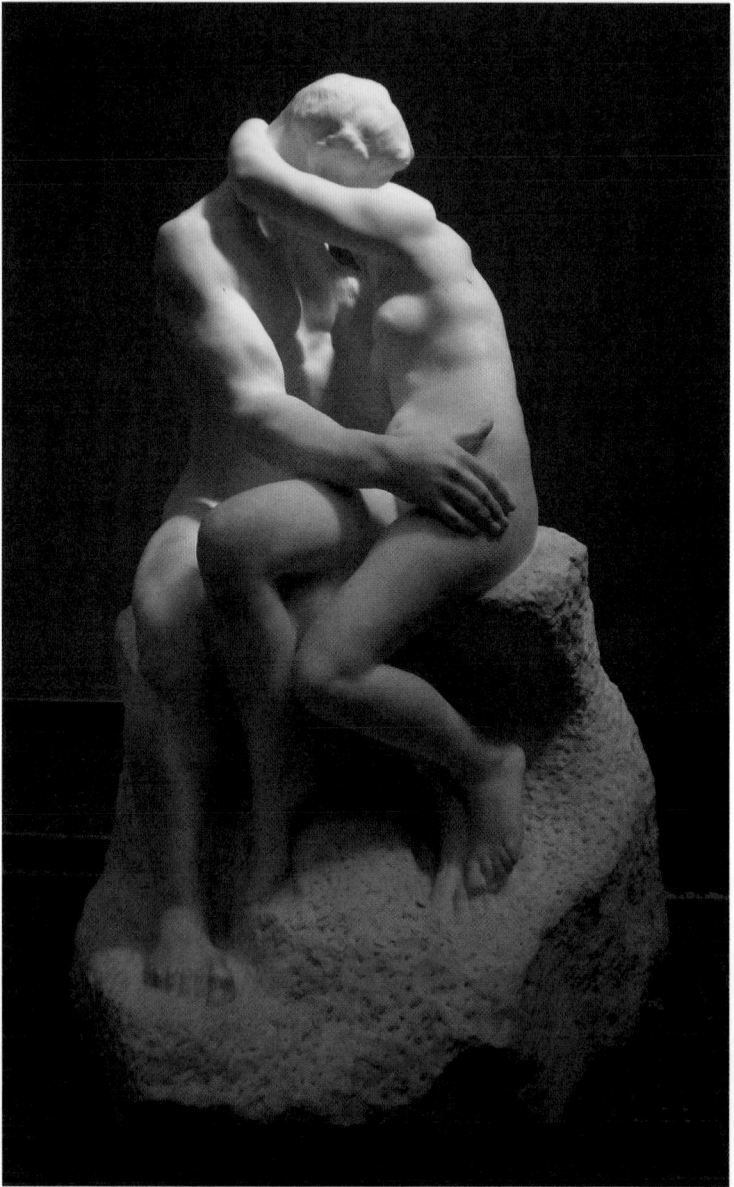

Auguste Rodin, *The Kiss*, 1901–4, marble.

Introduction:
Sex, Myth and Prehistory

T HE HUMAN SPECIES is at least partially defined by its ability to
conceive of the relationship between past, present and future.
Humans create plots – narratives with beginnings, middles and ends.
A significant aspect of our plot-making is sex, and sex is as important in our myths as it is in our lives. Myths are our cultural dreams,
and since the beginning of time we have dreamed of sex. Myths, of
course, also reflect other aspects of our existence, such as the need
to understand how we and our world came into being and how we fit
into the structure of the universe. But sex is pervasive in all mythologies because sex has obsessed us and confused us like no other
element of our individual and social being. The very fact that for
humans sex lies outside of the boundaries of the oestrus cycle that
regulates the sexuality of other mammals makes our sexual appetite
a central factor in our social existence, our rules of behaviour and,
by extension, our myth-making.

As early as the Upper Paaeolithic period, humans were depicting their fixation with sex in paintings on cave walls and with sexual
objects made of stone, bone or ivory. Archaeologists Marcos García-
Díez and Javier Angulo, students of this 'primitive' erotic art, go so
far as to suggest that 'the sexual appetite conditions humans as a
species'.

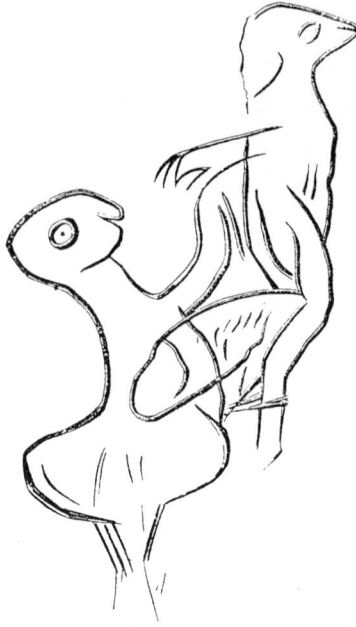

One of the earliest depictions of human coitus;
cave of Los Casares, Spain, c. 40,000 BCE.

Whether the drawings of male and female genitals, hetero- and homosexual copulation and other sex acts were related to prehistoric myths is, of course, open to question. What the art – even if some scholars dismiss it as mere graffiti – does make clear is that from at least 40,000 years ago humans were fixated on sex as something more than a function of reproduction. Several scholars – Joseph Campbell, Jamake Highwater, Sarah Dening and Marija Gimbutas among them – have centred their attention on several hundred tiny female figurines found in various sites in Europe, Anatolia and elsewhere, to argue that there was, in fact, a sexual Palaeolithic and Neolithic mythology based on fertility and female power. Among the most famous of these figurines are the Palaeolithic 'Venuses' of Willendorf in Austria, Hohle Fels in Germany (40,000 BCE), Laussel (*c.* 25,000 BCE) in the Dordogne region of France, and the Neolithic seated 'goddess' of the Anatolian Asia Minor site at Çatal Hüyük (*c.* 7500 BCE). These figurines have in common wide hips, huge breasts and vulvas in stylized triangles, all aspects suggesting sexuality and fertility and the dominance of the female in what these scholars see as matriarchal societies with female-based religions and associated myths in which sexuality was celebrated rather than repressed.

The word 'myth' as used here requires examination, as does the word 'sex'. Mythology is the study of myth. Mythologies are the collected myths of cultures. But in common usage a myth is a generally held belief that rational standards have rendered false. It is a myth that walking under a ladder will bring bad luck. Around sexuality there are many myths of this sort. It is now generally accepted by medical science that the old beliefs that masturbation has a negative effect on the human brain or that menstrual blood is somehow unclean and dangerous are 'myths'. The term 'myth' is frequently

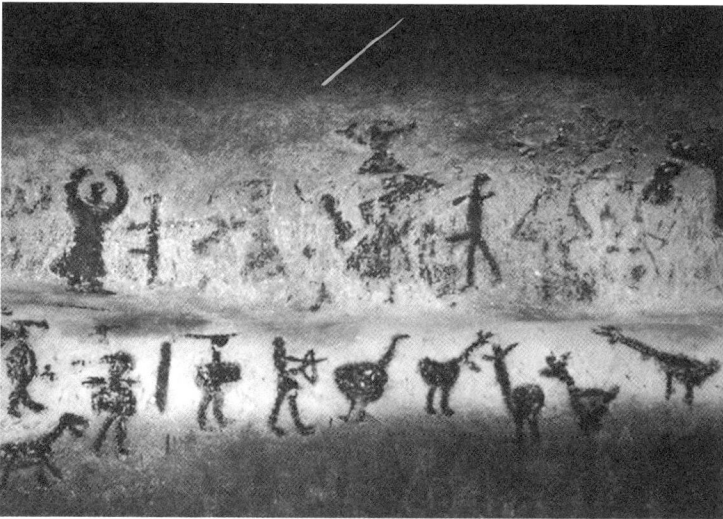

Erect hunters, Magura Cave, Bulgaria, *c.* 8000 BCE.

extended by scholars of various disciplines to refer to basic themes that pervade cultures or humanity in general, including the relationship between the genders. Thus the 'myth' of male superiority has informed most of the world's cultures for millennia. Few would deny that we still live in a patriarchal world today.

While these uses of 'myth' are valid enough, the precise meaning of the word comes from the Greek *mythos*, meaning 'story'. Mythos

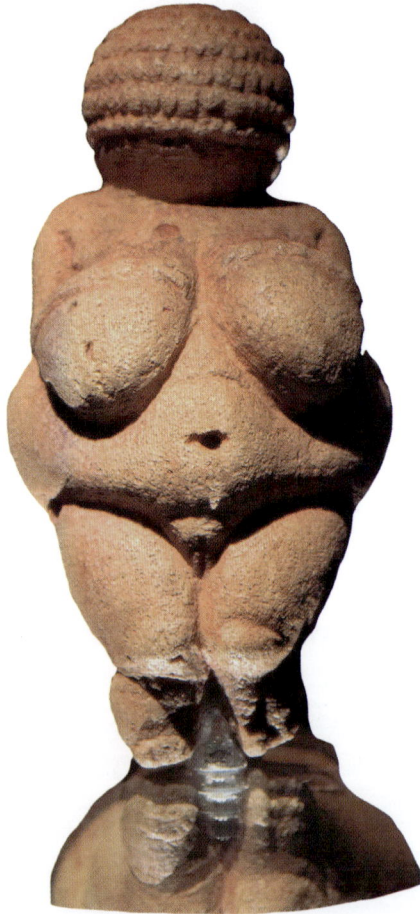

Venus of Willendorf, Austria, *c.* 25,000 BCE.

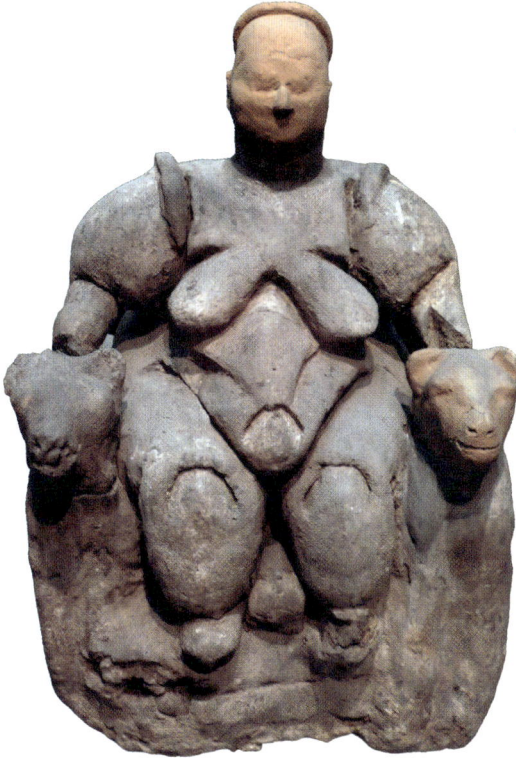

Venus of Çatal Hüyük, Turkey, *c.* 7500 BCE.

itself is derived from the original sound *mu*, denoting 'word'. A myth is a narrative which for many members of the culture that creates it might be literally or metaphorically 'true' while for others inside and outside of the culture it may be regarded as mere superstition – 'myth' in the sense of false belief described above. The story of the parting of the Red Sea contains a religious truth, whether literal or metaphorical for many Jews, Christians and Muslims. For Hindus or Buddhists it is simply a myth in the sense of a false – even if beautiful – story.

Myths always involve elements that transcend our ordinary experience of life. They emerge from the collective memories and suppositions of cultures. As cultural dreams, myths, even if literally untrue, reflect something of a culture's sense of itself and its preoccupations – such as sex.

'Sex' as used here refers to sexual acts described in myths or mythic images from around the world. The list of such acts includes vaginal intercourse, anal intercourse, oral sex, rape, bestiality, incest, masturbation and any number of acts one might find in a list of 'categories' on a pornographic Internet site. These acts can involve gods, goddesses or humans in various combinations and positions. The acts can be heterosexual or homosexual. They can involve transgender or hermaphroditic individuals. Certain themes are more prevalent in some cultures than in others. Penis length is a popular subject, as is ejaculation, contact between men and much younger women, and the sense that sexual acts can serve as a means of punishing women. Sex in mythologies can, of course, reflect cultural attitudes towards sexuality and gender in general. Myths can express, for instance, a male–female struggle in the sexual context. Myths such as those of Samson and Delilah or Medea and Jason reflect male anxiety about the power women can have over men in sexual relations – power that can be mitigated by male dominance in the sexual act itself and, by extension, in the larger social context.

Sexual myths, like all myths, can have many purposes. The reproductive acts of the ancient Greek goddess Gaia perhaps reflect a pre-Olympian matriarchal social system. The story of the rape of Persephone can explain the natural phenomena we call spring. The stories of the unbridled sexual deeds of the Polynesian Maui, the Native American Coyote and many other tricksters, as well as those of deities such as Aphrodite and Zeus, speak to a natural fascination with the power and mystery of sexual drives. Such myths can surely also have been meant to elicit laughter or titillation. Even when comic or prurient, however, the participation of sacred heroes – human incarnations of divine power – and deities, means that sexual myths are in some sense religious, pre-scientific partial answers to, or commentaries on, the nature of existence in general, and on both proper and improper acts of human sexuality in particular.

Michel Foucault, Mary Douglas and other scholars deny or de-emphasize the inherent importance of 'natural' genital-based appetites as the basis of sexuality, insisting that sexuality can only be understood in its cultural and historical context. From this perspective, for instance, the myth of the inherent difference between the sexes and assumed male dominance is based not on any inherent biology but is itself the result of cultural forces. This is why we have the existence of varying attitudes towards and rules regarding sex in cultures around the world. A study of sexual myths will naturally shed light on the essence of cultures. But if it is true that it is our attitude towards sex that differentiates us from other mammals and ultimately, therefore, in part defines us as a species, these myths must have a more general significance. Our varied cultural dreams about sexual acts, when viewed collectively, can provide insight into the psychology of the human species. The assumption here is that the human mind's struggle through its collective dreams to understand or to control the sexual appetite is fundamental to our understanding of who we are. A world tour of sexual myths is a good place to begin.

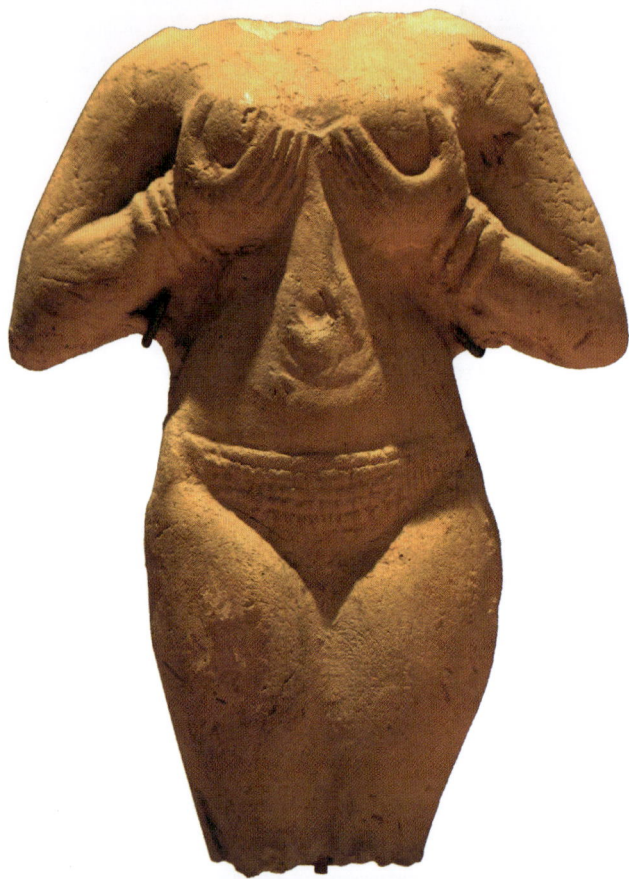

Female statuette, probably of the goddess Inanna,
thought to be Elamite, 3rd millennium BCE.

One

Mesopotamia

A T VARIOUS TIMES in the prehistoric period, myths came into being and were articulated not only in paintings and carved objects but in more developed form through oral transmission. Myths only enter the world of history, however, when they also find a written voice. Writing systems such as those found in Mesopotamia, Egypt and the Indus Valley gradually developed over the centuries from the primitive accounting tools of the late fourth millennium BCE into phonetically based systems suitable for storytelling in the third millennium. It is generally believed that the history of the literature of written myths began in southern Mesopotamia (now southern Iraq) among the people we call the Sumerians.

The Sumerians were a non-Semitic people who dominated southern Mesopotamia in several highly organized city-states in the fourth millennium BCE until they were gradually overcome by Semitic peoples beginning with the Akkadians under Sargon the Great in the middle of the third millennium. The Akkadian dominance of Mesopotamia was followed briefly by a resurgence of the Sumerians and then by conquests by other Semites – the Babylonians and the Assyrians. The Sumerian writing system, known as cuneiform (from the Latin *cuneus* for 'wedge' and *forma* for 'shape'), consisting of symbols wedged into little boxes on clay tablets, remained popular in Mesopotamia long after the Sumerians no longer existed as a people, and the myths that illustrated the Sumerian religion were adapted by the Mesopotamian dynasties that followed them, particularly by the Akkadians and Babylonians, into their own religious systems.

In the earliest Mesopotamian written myths involving sex acts, several characters central to the Sumerian religion stand out. These are Enki, the trickster god of wisdom, Inanna (later Ishtar), the great goddess of love, her husband Dumuzi (Tammuz) and the great hero-king Gilgamesh (Bilgamesh).

The Sumerian creation includes what would be a common motif in creation myths in many cultures, a motif which involves the necessary separation of the otherwise never-ending sexual intercourse between primeval parents. Here the union of Heaven (An) and Earth (Ki) resulted in the gods (the Anunnaki), who understood that their parents would have to be separated to make space for further creation. It was the couple's son, Enlil, later the head god, who took his mother away from the sky and established her as Earth. Enlil's most famous sibling was Enki, a half-brother whose father was An and whose mother was Nammu, the personification of the primeval sea, also known as 'Lady Vulva'.

Enki was the patron god of Eridu in what we now know as the marshlands of southern Iraq. He was a trickster, a god of magic and cunning. He lived in the Abzu, the fresh underground waters, and was associated with fertility, an identification which becomes clearer when we understand that in the Sumerian language 'water' and 'semen' were the same word. Rain, for instance, was the semen of An. Like tricksters from other cultures, Enki's sexual drive was insatiable and his phallus filled all the ditches of the marshland with his water (semen).

Enki was married to Damgalnuna ('True Wife'), one of many versions of the Mother Goddess. But Enki 'directed his semen . . . into the womb' of another Mother Goddess, Ninhursaga. Ninhursaga gave birth to the beautiful Nimmu, and Enki had incestuous intercourse with his daughter. When the goddess Ninkurra ('Mistress of the Land') was born of this relationship Enki had relations with her too, and produced Uttu ('Vegetation'). When Enki desired Uttu, Ninhursaga intervened, advising her great granddaughter to resist the god until he could provide her with apples, cucumbers and grapes. This Enki did and Uttu took him happily 'to her lap'. Ninhursaga then wiped excess semen from the girl's body and created eight new plants from the sacred fluid. To name these plants Enki ate them, an act that so enraged Ninhursaga that she cursed the god, bringing him close to death and turning the marshland into desert. Enki might have died, in fact, but for a little fox, who found a way of bringing the two deities back together. Ninhursaga then cured Enki by 'fixing' him 'in her vulva', presumably his proper place as a fertility god. It is this position that perhaps explains the god's name: *en-ki*, 'Lord [*en*] of Earth', Ninhursaga being an incarnation of the original Earth Goddess, Ki.

In terms of mytho-logic, it is evident that all the goddesses mentioned above, from Nammu to Uttu, are personifications of the concept of the great Mother Goddess, the Earth Mother who receives the seed of the fertility god Enki. The incest as described here becomes not so much a moral issue as a means of emphasizing specifically the importance of irrigation in the marshlands and more generally fertility in all aspects of life. The struggle between Ninhursaga and Enki leads to the near death of the land. Only when the deities are reconciled, when Enki is fixed in the 'lap' of the Great Earth Mother, is life possible.

The only Sumerian deity who rivalled Enki in popularity was Inanna, whose cult centre was Uruk (the biblical city of Erech from which Iraq perhaps takes its name). One of the most important Sumerian myths involves a culture-changing meeting between these two deities. The myth itself starts with a poignant sexual awakening scene in which the adolescent Inanna admires her genitals. Standing with her back against an apple tree in the sheepfold of the shepherd Dumuzi, who will later be her husband, she studies her vulva, her newly ripened sexuality. As author Diane Wolkstein translates the words of the myth, 'Rejoicing at her wondrous vulva, the young woman Inanna applauded herself.'

The anthropologist Gwendolyn Leick has suggested that in Sumer the apple tree was a common symbol for the male genitals. Gardens and other enclosures such as sheepfolds can serve similarly for the female genitals. It is not unreasonable to see masturbation as an element in this scene. In the sexual context, it is logical that immediately after admiring her new potentially productive and alluring self the young goddess decides that the time has come to visit Enki in the Abzu, the semen waters of Eridu.

Unlike in the myth of Enki and Ninhursaga, Enki resists any lustful feelings he might feel when the girl arrives in Eridu. Instead, he greets her with butter cakes and beer. The beer drinking becomes a contest; Enki and Inanna fill their cups to overflowing many times and Enki becomes so drunk that he offers the young goddess the sacred *me* of which he is guardian. The *me* are the universal laws that had emerged from Enki's mother, the primeval sea Mother, Nammu. They are the basis of Sumerian civilization – the standards of all activities: agricultural, political, social, familial and, of course, sexual. They include, for instance, the 'art of lovemaking', the 'art of prostitution', and even the art of 'kissing the phallus'. Inanna leaves with them safely stored in her boat – 'my vulva, the horn, the Boat of Heaven', as she will describe her 'boat' in the myth of her courtship of Dumuzi.

It is of interest that the powerful Enki loses control of the essence of Sumerian civilization – the *me* – to the goddess Inanna, the goddess of love. This myth perhaps reflects at least a remnant of the kind of Neolithic matriarchy hypothesized by Marija Gimbutas, Robert Graves and others. At the very least it speaks to the dominance of the love goddess during a period of Sumerian history. And with that dominance sex and religion came together and complemented each other as they rarely have in human culture.

Nowhere is this union of sex and religion more evident than in the story of Inanna and the shepherd Dumuzi. Returning to Uruk with the *me*, Inanna is now ready to take on her role as Queen of Earth. Later she will descend to the underworld to learn of death and infertility, but now she is poised to take on the role of Earth Goddess, the source of her land's fertility and life. As such she requires a seed bearer who will make her role possible. In the world of the goddess of love this means sex, pleasurable sex which, because of who she is, is religious sex.

Inanna's brother Utu, the sun god, looks down on his sister and reminds her that it is time to choose a husband. Will it be the farmer or will it be the shepherd? At first Inanna favours the farmer but later chooses the shepherd, Dumuzi, whose 'cream' and 'milk' are 'good' and who is more than willing to do the work of the farmer if the field to be farmed is Inanna. Dumuzi arrives at the young goddess's house with his cream and milk and calls out to his beloved to 'open the house' for him. Inanna's mother, who favours the marriage, commands her daughter to bathe and to anoint herself with oil. Then Inanna opens her door and the lovers 'press their necks together', a conventional term implying intimacy. What follows is a ritual dialogue between the lovers, a dialogue that reflects the Sumerian tradition of the sacred marriage in which the *en*, the king of the city, played the role of Dumuzi and a chosen woman, perhaps a priestess or sacred prostitute, that of Inanna.

In the myth, Inanna cries out that her vulva, the 'Boat of Heaven', is eager. She asks what are, in effect, liturgical questions: 'Who will plough my vulva . . . Who will plough my wet ground?' Dumuzi, now identifying himself as the king, provides the ritual answer: 'I, Dumuzi the king will plough your vulva.' Inanna then calls for the ploughing, and in Dumuzi's 'lap stood the rising cedar' and Inanna calls him 'my honey-man . . . my caresser of the soft thighs, the one my womb loves best.'

Dumuzi answers that he will 'drink' all the good things that Inanna's 'broad field' pours out – the products of their fertility. (It has been suggested by scholars that frequent depictions of women

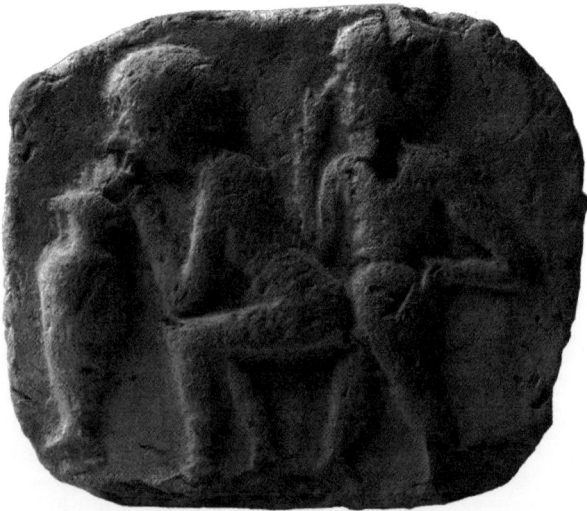

Drinking while loving: old Babylonian terracotta plaque, 3rd millennium BCE.

drinking during coitus was a convention to suggest fellatio. Men drinking during coitus might suggest cunnilingus.)

Continuing her conversation with Dumuzi the goddess calls on the king – now the 'wild bull' – to make his 'milk sweet and thick'. It is this 'fresh milk' that she will 'drink': 'Fill my holy churn with honey cheese.'

Later Inanna cries out that her 'priest' Dumuzi is ready for her 'holy loins', that his 'fullness' is her 'delight.' And Dumuzi 'filled my lap with cream and milk . . . stroked my pubic hair, laid his hands on my holy vulva . . . smoothed my black boat with cream.'

In turn, she will 'caress his loins' and he will use his mouth to please her – 'tongue-playing, one by one . . . fifty times.'

What is evident from these 'hymns' to Inanna, and from the physical example of Mesopotamian art recorded in clay and stone, is that sexuality of a particularly explicit sort was an important religious subject, tied, as in the Enki myths, to the fertility of the land. Enki's semen is the water that fertilizes the marshes. The result of sex between Inanna and Dumuzi is food: 'your broad fields pour out plants . . . grain . . . bread.' Inanna *is* the earth ploughed by the human 'king' Dumuzi. Sex is the natural metaphor for the agricultural process which pervaded the lives of the Sumerians and which they, like most cultures, saw as a cooperative venture between the divine and the human. There is no sense that sex is bad or best suppressed. Most importantly, there is no sense that the male is threatened by the power of the female's sexual drive. It is also evident, given the explicit imagery, that the scenes described are meant to be titillating. In the Sumerian world-view centred on the Great Goddess Inanna there is no conflict between titillation and religion.

There is, however, a hint of things to come, of what will become a power struggle between male and female – between the power of female sexual attraction and the male's drive for social position. After 'my sweet love is sated' Dumuzi begs Inanna to 'set me free . . . I would go to the palace', to begin cementing his position as king. When in another myth Inanna descends to the underworld to confront her 'dark side', sister Ereshkigal, and to learn the secrets of death, she leaves Dumuzi in charge of Uruk. Once in the underworld she is stripped of her power and effectively imprisoned. It is only with Enki's help that she escapes under a provision that a substitute for her must be sent to Ereshkigal. Inanna returns to Uruk after her three days in death to find Dumuzi not only not mourning her but enjoying his kingship and his new power. Enraged, she names her husband as her substitute in death, the planted seed without which the earth can no longer bear fruit. But Dumuzi's sentence is tempered when his sister agrees to spend half of each year in the underworld in his place, thus allowing Dumuzi to return to Uruk as king. This compromise with death is a theme that will emerge in the cultural dreams of other societies as well. In Greek myth, Alcestis, the wife of Admetus, sacrifices herself as a substitute in death for her brother. Anat does something similar for her brother, Baal, in Canaan, and in Egypt, Osiris' sister-wife turns her brother's death into a kind of resurrection. Implicit in these stories is the nature of the sexual relationship between the couples in question: Isis, to some extent Anat, and especially Inanna, are dominant figures who control their relationships, whereas Alcestis' heroic sacrifice signals sexual subservience. All are characters in a story that celebrates a return of sexual potency, itself signalling the fertility of the land.

By the end of the third millennium BCE the old Sumerian language had been displaced by the Semitic Akkadian language, even though the Akkadians, and the Babylonians and Assyrians, continued to use the Sumerian cuneiform script. The Semites also absorbed the old Sumerian mythology, but with adaptations and changes that fitted their own cultural priorities.

Sex in the Semitic adaptations of the Sumerian myths reflects a more warrior-oriented society and a male- rather than female-dominated, agriculturally based power structure. The change is particularly evident in the Babylonian creation story, the *Enuma Elish*, and in the Akkadian-Babylonian versions of what has become known as the *Epic of Gilgamesh*.

The *Enuma Elish* is, in effect, a revised creation story meant to celebrate an essential change. It tells the story of the emergence of Marduk, the warrior city god of Babylon, over the old gods and the former power of fertility goddesses. The old Sumerian mother goddess Nammu, the salt waters, has become the monstrous Tiamat. Her mate, Apsu, is a personification of the old fresh waters, the Sumerian Abzu. In the beginning Apsu had flowed sexually into the great mother and was absorbed by her greater power. This continual mating produced the old gods, one of the most important of whom was Ea, the Babylonian version of Enki. Ea's son was Marduk.

The gods quarrel with the original parents and Marduk agrees to lead a war in Heaven against Tiamat and Apsu but only if, after he defeats his adversaries, the gods promise to name him their sovereign. Marduk defeats the old Mother Tiamat and makes a new world out of the fragments of her body. His rule thereafter bears no resemblance to that of the Sumerian Inanna. His is a Zeus-like rule of male dominance.

In the Semitic pantheons, Inanna has become Ishtar, a goddess of war and, especially, of love, the forerunner of the later goddesses such as Astarte and Aphrodite. But as a love goddess she is no longer the earth to be ploughed and planted for fertility. She is, more than anything, a femme fatale, the epitome of the female power that threatens the independence and physical dominance of men. She is the mythological mother of Delilah, Medusa, Jezebel and Helen of Troy, those women who, in their sexual web, deprive men, at least temporarily, of their judgement and their public strength. Traditionally, in our predominantly patriarchal cultures, the way to combat such women has been to look the other way – as Perseus would do to avoid Medusa's deadly gaze – or to control their allure by depriving them of social power, by establishing socially approved mechanisms whereby women are owned by men. The Ishtar of the *Epic of Gilgamesh* is a remnant of the earlier age when she suggests to the hero Gilgamesh that they marry. But the Gilgamesh of the Semites knows better than to place himself under the spell of the love goddess. Instead of becoming a victim of seduction Gilgamesh defies her.

The Gilgamesh story, of course, has its roots in the oral and written traditions of Sumer, but the versions we know have come to us via Akkad and Babylon and are deeply influenced by the traditions of those cultures. In an ancient Sumerian tale known as *The Huluppu Tree*, Gilgamesh is a king of Uruk who comes to the aid of Inanna by reclaiming the sacred tree she hopes will supply the wood for her throne. The tree has been invaded by three lawless figures. These are the Anzu Bird, which had once tried to steal the sacred *me* from Enki, the evil woman whom we know as Lilith, and the snake, the ancestor of the serpent who appears in the Garden of Eden tree. Gilgamesh in this story comes to Inanna's rescue, kills the snake and expels the other intruders. He cuts down the tree so that it can be used by Inanna as her throne, the symbol of her dominance in Sumer, and as her bed, the place of her productive lovemaking celebrated in the sacred marriages between Uruk kings and the priestesses or holy prostitute-representatives of the goddess.

Gilgamesh here is the sacred king, the representative, like Dumuzi, of the union between Uruk and its goddess.

In the Gilgamesh epic, when Ishtar approaches Gilgamesh with her proposal, there is no indication of the old relationship between them. Gilgamesh is with his companion Enkidu and immediately refuses the goddess's offer of sex. The friendship with Enkidu represents the idea of male companionship as somehow superior to the sex-drugged relationship of men with women. Enkidu has been sent to Uruk by the mother goddess Ahuru (Sumerian Nammu) to counteract the king's wrongful claiming of a *droit de seigneur* with the newly wed women of his city. Enkidu arrives as an animal man, but Gilgamesh hears of him and sends a sacred prostitute to tame him for civilized life. The woman 'bared her breast' to Enkidu and treated him to a ritual six days and nights of ardent lovemaking. Once 'civilized', at least in the old Sumerian sense, Enkidu challenges Gilgamesh to a wrestling match, a match which Gilgamesh eventually wins. After that the two men embrace and vow eternal friendship. When Enkidu dies after the heroes kill a monster sacred to some of the gods, Gilgamesh is distraught and literally goes to the ends of the earth in search of eternal life and, by extension, Enkidu. There have been suggestions that the Gilgamesh-Enkidu relationship is homosexual, much as there have been suggestions about the Patroclos-Achilles relationship in the *Iliad*. When first presented with Enkidu, Gilgamesh is told he would love him 'like a wife'.

Whatever the nature of their relationship, their treatment of Ishtar is collective and violent. When the goddess asks him to sow his seed in her, Gilgamesh reminds her of the many victims of her charms, including Tammuz (Dumuzi) who now spends half of each year in the underworld because of her, and he points out that he knows he will be discarded when her desire is sated. Furious at his

Gilgamesh and
Enkidu – wrestling
or loving? Old
Babylonian
clay tablet.

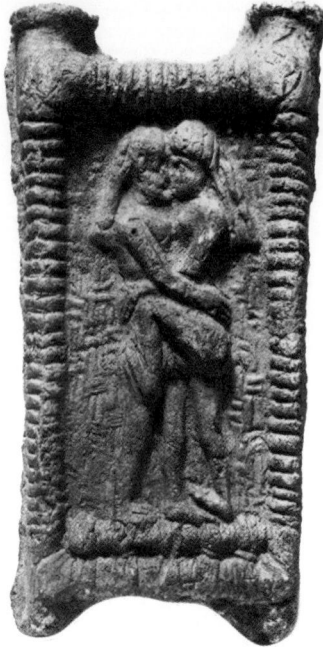

refusal, Ishtar arranges for the Bull of Heaven, the old traditional
consort of the Great Goddesses of Çatal Hüyük and other Neolithic
sites, to come to her aid. But the heroes slay the bull and fling its
bloody haunch at the now hysterical and un-Inanna-like Ishtar.

The cultural distance between the Sumerian hymns of Inanna
and the story of the insult to Ishtar is significant; it involves two rad-
ically different attitudes towards human sex. Inanna's sexuality was
natural and fertility-based, whereas the sex of her Semitic incarnation,
Ishtar, is dangerous and threatening to male power. This emergence
of femme fatale sexuality stands as a representative moment in world
mythology. It will play out in later mythologies in which heroes and
nations are threatened by the sexual power of women such as Morgan
le Fay and Helen of Troy.

Two

Egypt

As civilization developed in Mesopotamia, another great culture was emerging in Egypt. In what is known as the Early Dynastic period, at the end of the fourth millennium BCE, the Egyptians, like the Sumerians, had created a writing system. We know this system as hieroglyphics (Greek: 'sacred script') in which pictorial symbols represented ideas, sounds or words. Supposedly invented by the god Thoth, hieroglyphics only became understandable to the post-Egyptian world with the discovery in 1799 of the so-called Rosetta Stone, on which appeared a royal decree written in hieroglyphs, demotic Egyptian and Greek, making a translation of the hieroglyphs by comparison possible. Egyptian myths have come to us from Greek writers such as Herodotus, Diodorus Siculus and Plutarch, but their understandings of the myths are deeply coloured by their tendency to force a somewhat simplistic relationship between mythic figures of Egypt with those of Greece. Among the most important primary sources for Egyptian mythology are the *Pyramid Texts* of the mid-third millennium BCE, and the *Coffin Texts* of the late third millennium BCE. These were accounts and spells (funerary texts) carved into the walls of tombs. Over the centuries, myths were also recounted in collections such as the mid-second millennium *Book of the Dead* and other papyrus texts. The *Pyramid Texts* and *Coffin Texts* reflected the theology of the most prominent of the Egyptian religious centres, that of Heliopolis, near present-day Cairo. Sex plays an important role in this theology, beginning with a creation myth.

As in the case of many creation myths, existence rises in Egypt out of the chaotic primeval waters. In this case a mound – the *benben* – rises out of the waters (*Nun*) as the place on which the creator god Atum will sit. Atum later is Atum-Ra, the sun emerging from the darkness represented by the *benben*. Some texts interpret the *benben* as the petrified semen of Atum. Replicas of the *benben* formed the tips of the great pyramids and Egyptian obelisks. The obvious phallic implications of the *benben*, pyramids and obelisks are supported by the Heliopolis creation myth.

Sitting on the mound, the god, known as the 'Complete One', or by some as the 'Great He-She', can only create from himself. This he does by masturbation, using his female aspect, the 'Hand of Atum', sometimes personified as the great mother goddess Hathor, the celestial cow on whose horns the sun rests in Egyptian iconography. In the *Pyramid Texts* Atum identifies himself by his creative act: 'I am he who rubbed with his fist, I emitted into my own hand.' In some understandings of the myth, Atum swallows his semen, an act of autofellatio by which he becomes literally mother and father to his progeny, later sneezing out the god Shu (Air) and spitting out the goddess Tefnut (Moisture).

Atum identifies Shu further as the life force (*ka*) and Tefnut as the ordering logos of life (*maat*). The first mating between a male (Shu) and a female (Tefnut) – an incestuous mating of the life force and essential order – justifies metaphorically the incestuous mating of pharaohs and their sisters and, given the representation of the two gods as *ka* and *maat*, perhaps suggests an Egyptian ideal of the nature of males and females and their places in society.

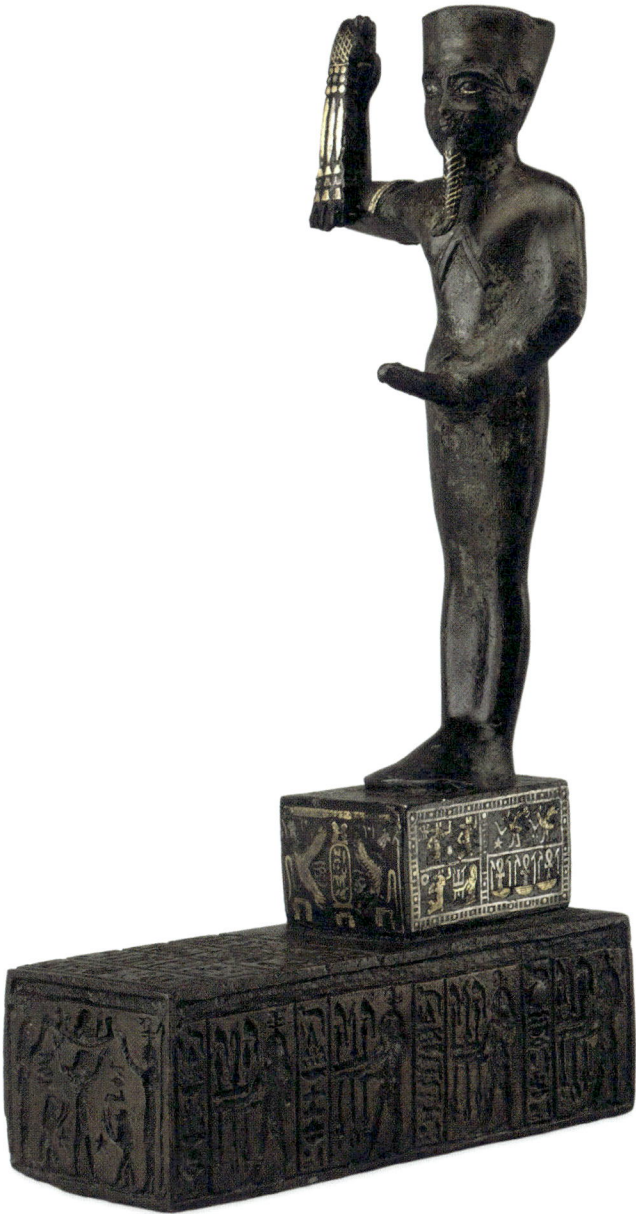

Erect creator god, bronze statue, 7th century BCE.

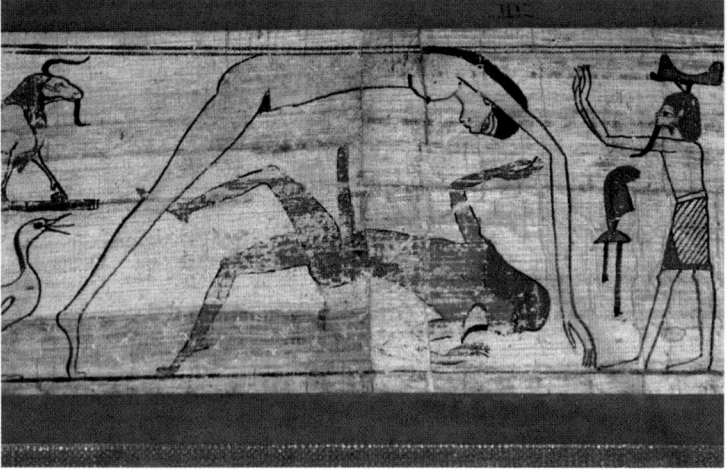

Geb and Nut, depicted on the *Papyrus of Tanienu, c.* 1000 BCE.

Tefnut gave birth to a son, Geb (Earth), and a daughter Nut (Sky), reversing the usual order in other mythologies of the male as the sky god and the female as the Earth Goddess. Scholars have suggested that this fact indicates an Egyptian tendency to favour the female-on-top position in intercourse. Whatever their chosen positions in their first days, Geb and Nut made love continually without concern for anything else, leaving no room between them (Sky and Earth) for further creation. Clearly, separation was called for. In Sumer, An and Ki (Sky and Earth) were separated by their son. Here it falls to Shu (Air, the life force), the father of the lovers, to separate the primeval parents and hold them apart, even as Geb strains to regain connection with his sister-spouse. Geb is often depicted in a prone position beneath her with an exaggerated erection that itself suggests an obelisk.

A late manuscript tells how Geb resented his father's role in the separation and that in revenge he separated Shu from Tefnut and either raped his mother or made her his queen. This tale adds

34

little to the original Heliopolis myth, but it is of interest because it coincides with stories of father-son rivalries and sexual taboos in other mythologies. Greek mythology, for instance, begins with the struggles between the god Ouranos and his son Kronos and between Kronos and his son Zeus. And at the centre of both of those rivalries is what the modern world would see as the Freudian relationship between the mother and her son who stand together against the father.

After the separation of Geb and Nut, their conceived children can be born. These children, Osiris, his sister-wife Isis, Seth (Set) and his sister-wife Nephtys, in addition to Atum, Shu, Tefnut, Geb and Nut, form the Heliopolis pantheon of nine primary gods known as the Ennead. The four younger gods with the still younger Horus, child of Osiris and Isis, are the primary players in a sex-laced drama that is at the centre of Egyptian mythology.

Osiris, the oldest of Geb and Nut's children, ruled Egypt in a golden age. Many sexual myths about Osiris emerged over time, one even claiming that he first had intercourse with Isis in their mother's womb. Another tale relates how Nephtys, whose husband Seth was, apparently, sterile, tricked Osiris into having sex with *her*, resulting in the god Anubis, the dog-headed god of the afterlife and mummification. Either the discovery of his brother's relationship with his wife or, according to a *Pyramid Text*, resentment because Osiris had once kicked him, led Seth to turn against his brother. Seth killed Osiris, either by drowning or dismembering him, or both. Osiris was mourned deeply by Isis, who searched the world or the Nile for his body parts. According to Plutarch, the penis was the only irretrievable part because it had been eaten by a fish. In some versions Isis made models of the penis and buried them or the other body parts along the Nile, effectively fertilizing the land so that Osiris, now dead, but king of the underworld, became a central fertility deity, his planted parts rising each year from the flood as food. A *Coffin Text* equates Osiris with grain: 'I am the plant of life, which grows from the ribs of Osiris / which allows the people to live.' Apparently, at certain festivals the phallus of Osiris was carried in procession to celebrate that fertility. Mythologically it seems clear that the

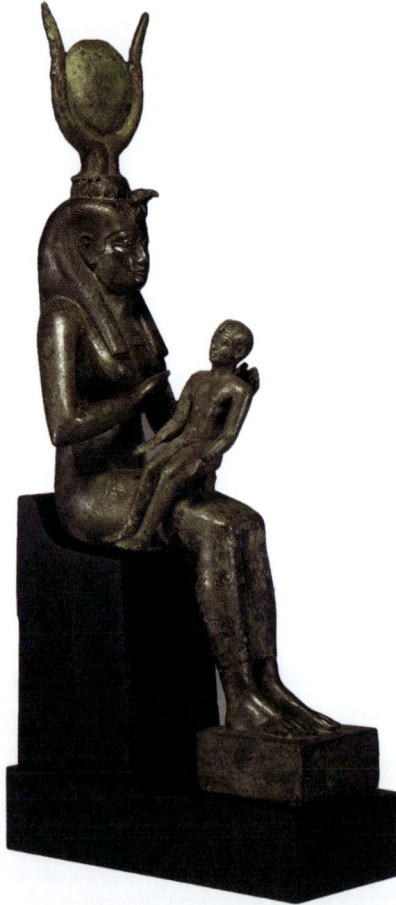

Isis nursing the baby Horus, bronze statue,
Alexandria, 4th century CE.

.

Seth-Osiris conflict represents a constant struggle between infertility and fertility, death and life, itself enacted in the annual death of the land in the Nile flood-waters followed by its fertile resurrection as the waters receded. Later, Christians would celebrate a similar pattern in the rite of Baptism, in which the initiate 'dies' to his or her spiritually infertile past-life in the waters of the font and is reborn into a new spiritually fertile life with Christ.

In all versions of the Osiris myth, Isis emerges as the central figure. She and her sister Nephtys perform mourning rituals over the dead body of Osiris in hopes of reviving him. Revival is necessary because Isis has been told that she will conceive a child who will be king. Geraldine Pinch points out a connection here to the role of the 'Hand of Atum' in the original creation. In effect Isis becomes that hand as she takes the form of a bird and flutters over her husband to arouse him so that the child Horus, the future king, representing a new creation, can be conceived.

Fearing Seth, who is now king in Osiris' place, Isis flees Upper Egypt in favour of a hidden place in the marshes of the Delta to give birth to her child. This place, a papyrus grove on an island in the marshes, became known as the 'nest of Horus'. There the child is nursed by his mother, who sometimes takes the form of the cow goddess Hathor, who had personified the 'Hand of Atum' in the old creation and was now nurturing this new one. It is impossible to ignore certain likenesses to the Christian nativity story here and to the story of the baby Moses hidden in the bull rushes.

The young Horus is threatened by Seth, but as he grows he is determined to wrest the kingship from his murderous uncle. Seth is equally determined to maintain his position. When poison and other methods fail to eliminate Horus, he turns to sex. The boy Horus reveals to his mother that Seth has been admiring his buttocks and wishes to sleep with him. Isis advises her son to agree to do so only in return for some of the older god's magical power. Seth agrees, but Isis also commands her son to capture Seth's semen in his hand. This Horus does and returns to his mother, who cuts off his hand and throws it into the river before making the boy a new hand. She now acts once again as the 'Hand of Atum' by masturbating her son and capturing some of his semen. This semen she spreads on some of Seth's favourite lettuce plants. When Seth eats the lettuce, he becomes pregnant and gives birth to the sun disc which the god Thoth places on Horus' head, proclaiming him the true son of the sun God.

In another version of this story, Seth eats the lettuce as described above, not realizing that it contains Horus' semen. He attempts to shame Horus and undermine his claims to the throne by exposing him as a passive homosexual in a council of the gods. He claims to the gods that his semen is within Horus' body. A late second millennium BCE text reveals something of the reaction of ancient Egyptians to at least one aspect of homosexual sex. The gods 'cried out and spat at Horus' in disgust. But Horus denies the charge and challenges the gods to produce the semen. When the god Thoth commands the semen to come out it comes out from Seth's body rather than Horus'. Humiliated, Seth leaves the council and Horus' honour remains intact. This story assumes a common belief among ancient and modern people in various parts of the world that homosexual sex is demeaning, but only to the individual penetrated.

In the battle between Seth and Horus, Horus loses his eye and Seth his testicles. Seth's tearing apart of the eye and Horus' castration of Seth point back to the mutilation of Osiris. The battle between Seth and Horus so disturbs the universe that Atum and the other gods put a stop to it, deciding that Horus should be king.

Seth loses power and fertility with the tearing out of his testicles. Horus' lost eye is equivalent to Atum's eye and to the sun; it is light itself. As Horus becomes king, the eye is reassembled and restored, as Osiris had been, and becomes the Udjat (Wedjat), the symbol of pharaonic power and legitimacy. With the literal and metaphorical rise to power of Horus, the pattern or divine order is finally established whereby all Egyptian kings die as Osiris and are born as the sexually potent Horus.

An indication of Horus' new power – specifically his virility – is his association in the second millennium BCE with the ithyphallic god Min as Min-Horus. Min was celebrated particularly at coronations, when the king was supposed to literally produce the seed of life which would ensure the annual flooding of the Nile. In so doing he would repeat the masturbatory act of Atum in creation itself. The seed metaphor is expressed frequently in temple art in which an isolated erect phallus is depicted ejaculating drops of semen.

An example of the emphasis on this metaphor exists also in an image of King Tutankhamun sitting with his bow while his queen sits at his feet holding an arrow. Given the fact that in the Egyptian language 'shoot' also meant 'ejaculate', this image has been widely interpreted to refer to the ritual ejaculation of the pharaoh in relation not only to the rising of the flooding Nile but to a belief that sex was a necessary element of the passage to the afterlife, the central concern of Egyptian myth and ritual. This association refers to the sex act between the dead Osiris and his wife Isis before Osiris descended to the underworld to become king there.

If the sexual mythology of the Sumerians was vulva-centric, then, that of the ancient Egyptians, framed by the masturbatory acts of Atum and Min, was clearly phallocentric. It is worth noting in this connection what seems to have been an early example of the

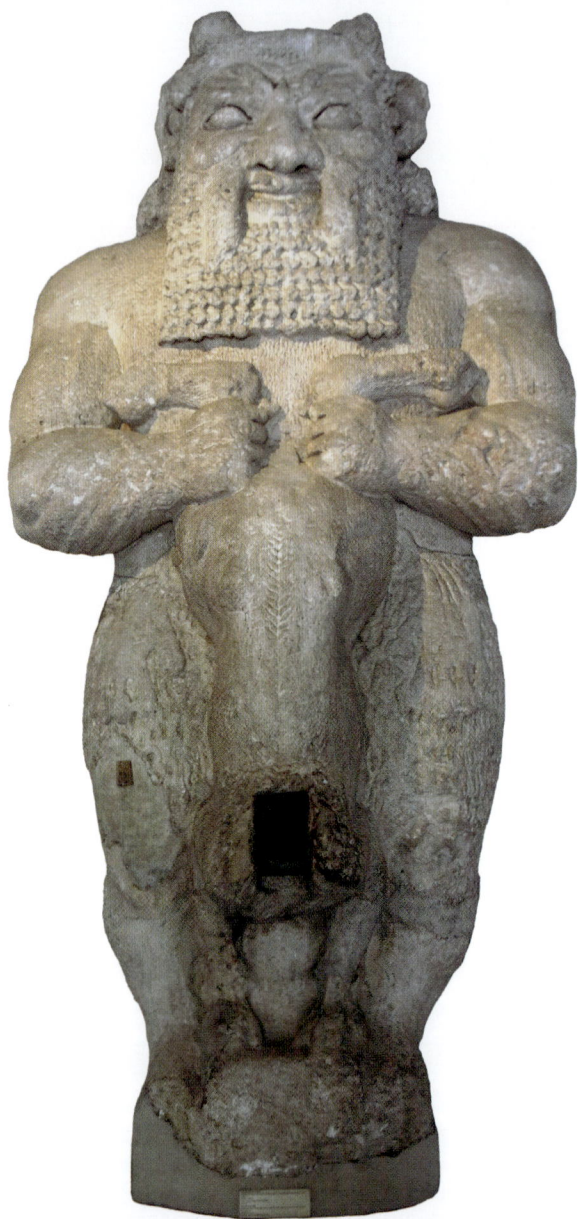

Limestone statue of half-god Bes, 1st century CE.

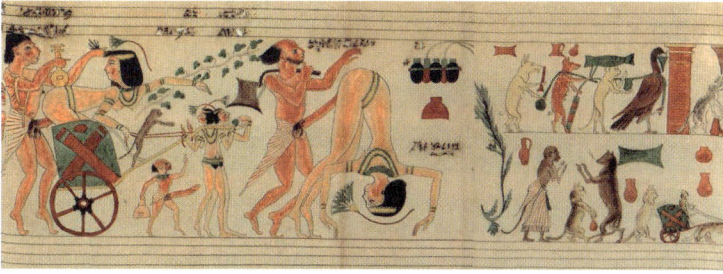

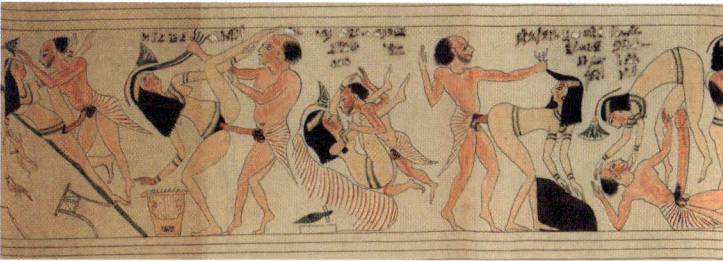

Reconstruction of the *Turin Erotic Papyrus*, an Egyptian scroll, *c*. 1100 BCE.

human tendency to be fascinated by penis size. The god Bes, who was associated with fertility, sensual pleasure and the power to ward off evil, was often depicted sporting a large phallus and appears to have been primarily a comic figure.

This comic fascination with the penis is also evident in the so-called Turin Erotic Papyrus, a fragmented papyrus found at Deir el-Medina containing explicit depictions of sexual activities. The papyrus dates from about 1100 BCE. Whether these depictions are early examples of pornography intended to titillate or elicit laughter or some sort of mythological representation is unclear. What does clearly dominate the papyrus is phalli of exaggerated size such as would be found later in the art of China, Japan, Greece, Rome and elsewhere, as well as in the pornography of all cultures.

This nearly universal fascination with the penis and penis size in 'art' devised by men indicates a perception of the penis as a weapon

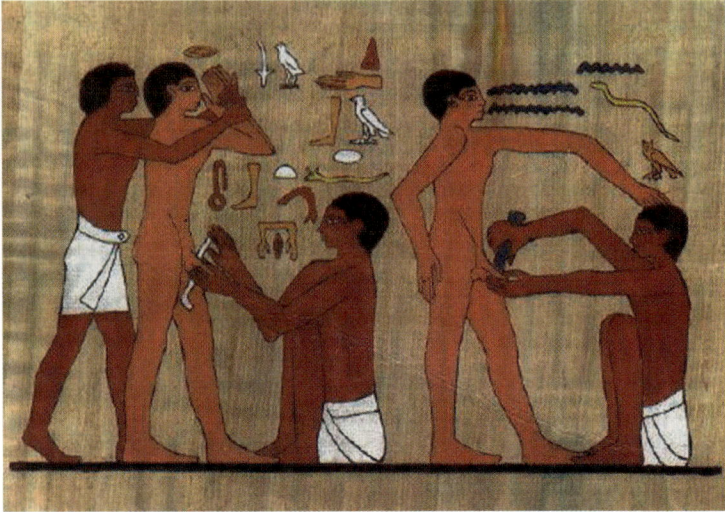

Egyptian circumcision depicted in a tomb painting, Sakhara, 2350–2000 BCE.

rather than as an instrument of love or even procreation. The porno-graphically enlarged penis is a weapon, allowing the man to assert his control over the woman. The size of the penis becomes a primary sign of manliness, dominance and power and expresses a sense of gender relations that is very different from that expressed in the Sumerian Inanna hymns or in the 'Song of Songs' in the Bible.

Another example of the fixation on the penis in Egypt was the practice of circumcision, which possibly originated there. The hiero-glyphic symbol for 'penis' was the erect or the circumcised member. The reason for the practice of circumcision is not known. There are several possibilities, including cleanliness, a symbol of status, a ritual indicating passage from childhood to adulthood, or, as in the neigh-bouring Hebrew culture, a divine command.

Three

Canaan and Israel

A LATE EGYPTIAN GODDESS borrowed from the Canaanites is Qetesh. She was often represented in Egypt standing between the ithyphallic Min and the war god Resheph. Like many Middle Eastern goddesses of love and sexuality she is also a patroness of war and warriors. Love is rarely one-sided, she seems to say, as she presents the lotus flower of desire to Min and the snake of battle to her husband Resheph. As a representative of both sex and war, Qetesh is, in effect, a mythological sister to the Mesopotamian goddess Ishtar and the love and war goddesses of Canaan.

In ancient Canaan goddesses and their sexuality played a significant mythological role and stood in opposition to the emerging monotheistic patriarchal mythology of the Hebrews, who invaded much of their territory, a land the Hebrews would later proclaim to be the 'Promised Land', the land promised them by a god who recognized no goddesses.

The second millennium BCE had seen a flourishing of what we now call Canaanite centres in the land that encompasses present-day Israel, Palestine, Syria, Jordan and Lebanon. 'Canaanite' is a catch-all term referring to a variety of Semitic-speaking tribes in the area. Jebusites created what is now the city of Jerusalem. Ugaritics settled the city of Ugarit (Ras Shamra in modern Syria). Amorites lived

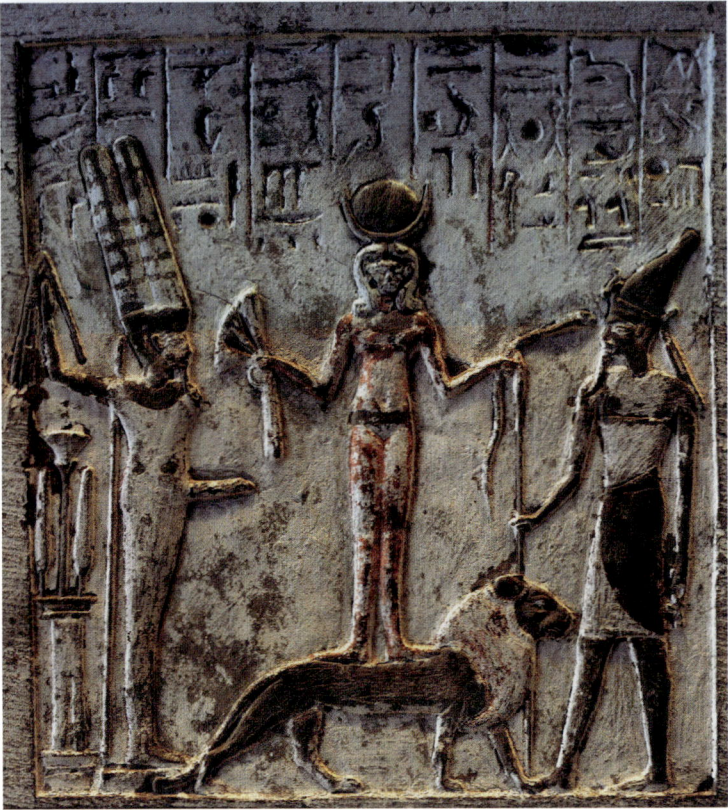

Qetesh, between the Egyptian god Min and the Canaanite god Resheph, stele, *c.* 1200 BCE.

in Mari on the border between modern Syria and Iraq. A group the Greeks called Phoenicians lived along the coast of what is now Lebanon.

The Phoenicians invented an alphabet to replace the old cunei-form script, making writing simpler and more efficient. Discoveries of written material, especially at sites in Phoenicia, Ugarit and Mari, have provided insight into Canaanite mythology, which was some-what influenced by that of the Mesopotamian Semites, and much of which was absorbed by the non-Semitic Philistines in what is now southern Palestine.

Hebrew mythology associates the Canaanites specifically with a sexual taboo involving the penis. In the Hebrew Bible (Genesis 9:20) Noah became drunk and was lying 'uncovered' in his tent when his son Ham, the father of Canaan, entered and witnessed his father's nakedness. Ham told his brothers, Shem and Japheth, what he had seen and they, with averted faces, went in to restore their father's modesty with a garment. When Noah woke up he somehow knew what had happened, and in a rage he cursed Ham's progeny, namely, Ham's son Canaan, who would be a slave to his relatives. Why was Canaan the target of the curse rather than Ham? In the Talmud (rabbinic commentaries on the Torah), various somewhat extreme explanations are offered. Did Ham perhaps castrate his father or at least metaphorically do so by seeing his genitals? Emasculation would have prevented Noah from having a fourth son. Thus, Ham's fourth son, Canaan, was cursed. Another Talmudic explanation is that Ham sodomized his father. It seems more likely that Ham literally broke sexual laws by seeing Noah's genitals. In the biblical Book of Leviticus Yahweh includes seeing one's father 'uncovered' among forbidden acts, although it must be pointed out that experiencing the uncovered father has been interpreted by some scholars to refer to having intercourse with the father. In any case, as the son had sinned, the sin would be passed on to the son's son. And so, in hindsight, the invasion of Canaan by the Hebrews would be justified in the Bible when it was written. The man Canaan was vile and so the people he represented became vile. The land of Canaan was associated with sexual sin.

Canaanite mythology, like that of the other civilizations in the Middle East, such as the Mesopotamians, the Egyptians and the

Hittites, was primarily concerned with the fertility of the land. In Canaan, gods and goddesses performed metaphorical roles reflecting the variations of seasons and weather patterns. The head of the Canaanite pantheon was El, whose Semitic name, meaning essentially 'the god', is a cognate for the Arab Semitic Allah (al-ilah) and the Hebrew Semitic Elohim (a plural of el but used as a singular noun). El, like his predecessor in Sumer, achieved power after overpowering – presumably dividing – his parents, Heaven and Earth. Until the emergence of Baal as the dominant god, El was the source of Canaanite life, the sky god who ensured the earth's fertility. An Ugaritic tablet describes a creation story in which El once stood on the seashore with his two wives or consorts, one of whom was the 'mother of Gods', Asherah, when his 'hand' – interpreted as 'penis' – grew to a great length, and he impregnated both women simultaneously, giving birth to dawn and dusk.

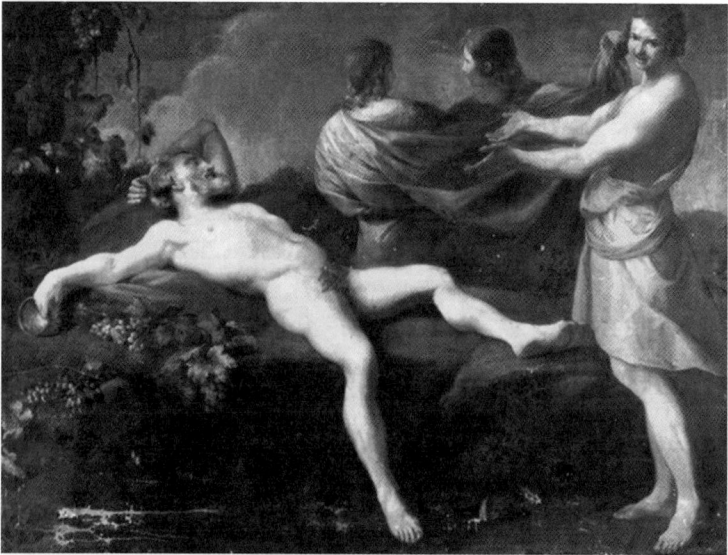

Andrea Sacchi, *Noah and his Sons*, 17th century, oil on canvas.

As was the case in Semitic Mesopotamia, where the old gods were supplanted by the Babylonian city god Marduk, and in Greece where Zeus would replace his father, El was reduced in importance in Canaanite mythology by the popular Ugaritic storm-weather god, Baal. Either the son of El or of Dagon, the god of grain, Baal went to war against the old gods, including those of the sea, and violent storms, the equivalents of Tiamat and Apsu in the *Enuma Elish*. After his victory he confronted Death (Mot or Yam), who had invited him to the underworld. Mot represents infertility, the opposite of Baal (life), who, before he departed for Mot's world, took the form of a bull – the preferred guise of most ancient fertility gods – and mated 88 times with a goddess who took the form of a heifer. That goddess is usually considered to have been his sister Anat, the 'virgin' goddess of love and war.

Baal's dangerous descent to Mot is analogous to the Sumerian Inanna's descent to the underworld ruled by her sister-opposite Ereshkigal, the embodiment of death and infertility. With Baal's absence the land died, but with Anat's help, reminiscent of Isis' revival of Osiris, Mot was defeated and Baal returned to Earth bringing back its fertility, a fact emphasized by his being sometimes depicted with characteristics of both sexes, both being required for gestation.

Annual ceremonies of the Baal cycle in Canaan celebrated the turn from winter to spring, from periods of drought to rain, from infertility to fertility. According to one theory the rite of *hieros gamos* was practised in these celebrations, a rite in which representatives of Baal and the virgin goddess Anat copulated to represent this fertility. This was a tradition similar to the one that took place in Sumer between the king representing Dumuzi and the sacred prostitute representing Inanna. Such practices were probably based on the idea that the gods – El and Asherah, Baal and Anat (or Asherah) – would be stimulated by the ritual to come together themselves, thus ensuring the fertility of the land.

Anat is one of several important goddesses in the Baal cycle and Canaanite mythology in general who collectively compose what is really a single goddess with many names. Asherah (or Ashtoreth, or Athirat), the 'Mother of Gods', begins as El's wife and then, in some texts, becomes Baal's. In Phoenicia Asherah is Astarte ('Baal's Other Self'), and Astarte, as a love-war goddess, is a cognate for Anat, and by association for the Canaanite-Egyptian Qetesh, the Babylonian Ishtar and the Egyptian Isis. Aspects of this combined goddess would become Aphrodite in Greece.

The goddess in various forms would challenge her male opposite in the minds of the semi-nomadic tribes we call Hebrews, who emerged as a significant power in Canaan in the late second millennium BCE. This was at about the time of the arrival of the Philistines in the area and of the Trojan War, if such a war took place. The details of the Hebrew emergence are shrouded in mystery, since the records we have of it are based on biblical mythology. This mythology is centred around a narrative that begins with the story of the patriarch Abraham and continues with those of his sons, Ishmael and Isaac, Isaac's son Jacob (renamed Israel), and Moses, who is said to have led the Hebrews (Israelites) from Egypt to the 'Promised Land'. The final versions of the biblical stories themselves – especially those of Genesis, Exodus and the other books forming the Torah, based on oral and written segments dating from the late second millennium BCE – were probably composed in Mesopotamia during the exile of Israelites there in the sixth century BCE and in Israel in the post-exilic period beginning in about 539 BCE.

There is some historical evidence that a king named David made Jebus – the city of the Jebusites, later Jerusalem – the capital of an Israelite state in the tenth century BCE and that his successor Solomon built the first temple to Yahweh there, but this evidence is inconclusive. What does seem likely is that the Hebrew tribes both fought for territory against and absorbed things from the Canaanites, learning writing from them, for instance, and adopting many of their religious traditions, which would have conflicted with the development of the monotheistic Yahweh religion which they perhaps learned originally from the Midianites, the tribe to which, according to tradition, Moses' wife belonged.

The Hebrew tribes who came to Canaan must have been impressed and drawn by the fertility of the land. And if Baal, the god worshipped by the Canaanites, was ascribed as the source of this fertility, it would certainly have been tempting to worship that god and his attending goddesses, as well as the old high god El. In the Torah, the deity introduced himself to Abraham as El Shaddai (El of the Mountain). Even Israelite rulers were tempted. King Ahab in the mid-ninth century BCE married the daughter of the King of Phoenicia, Jezebel, one of the many biblical femmes fatales. Under the queen's influence, he adopted the Baal religion and built a temple to the Canaanite god in his capital, Samaria. The fertility rites of the Canaanites were practised widely, including, for instance, the worship of the Canaanite collective goddess in the form of phallic stones known as Asherah poles. The prophets of the Yahweh religion resisted the Baal worship, including the suggestion that Asherah was Yahweh's wife. For them, Asherah was El's wife or Baal's. Yahweh's proper 'wife' was Israel. The Israelites were, in effect, committing adultery by consorting with the likes of Baal and Asherah. In fact, the creation of the written Torah and the elimination of de facto Israelite polytheism through the full establishment of the Yahweh religion – Judaism – would not take place until the Babylonian exile, followed by the eventual return to the 'Promised Land.'

In the mythology of Judaism, as contained in the Torah and the later books of the Bible (the Tanakh) and in the rabbinical commentaries and laws known as the Talmud, Asherah and related fertility cults may have been suppressed, but sex remained an important element in the biblical narrative, if even by its significant absence.

It all begins with Genesis, which, unlike the creation stories of Sumer, Egypt and Canaan, describes an *ex nihilo* (from nothing) creation in which the creating deity works asexually with no mate and no use of genitals. In Genesis 1, Yahweh does create a male human and a female human whom he urges to be 'fruitful'. Soon, in Genesis 2, sex comes more explicitly into the narrative, but in association with sin, not with fertility as in the older cults of the region. The Genesis 2 story of the creation of humans is different from that of Genesis 1. Here God creates the man – Adam – first and then the woman (womb-man?), Eve, from the man's rib. Both are naked but they do not recognize the concept of nakedness. This state of passionless purity in the Garden of Eden is undermined when Sàtan, in the form of the serpent, convinces the woman to eat fruit from the Tree of Knowledge forbidden them by the creator. The woman then entices her mate to do so, thus becoming the first in a long line of femmes fatales in the Bible. After eating the fruit, the couple attain 'knowledge', becoming aware of their nakedness, feeling shame and associating that shame with their genitals, which they cover with fig leaves. Thus, in the Western traditions developing from and deeply influenced by this myth, sex is related to an original sin, and women are established as the dangerous power behind that sin.

The supposedly dangerous aspect of women is emphasized in Jewish folklore in the person of Lilith, supposedly Adam's first

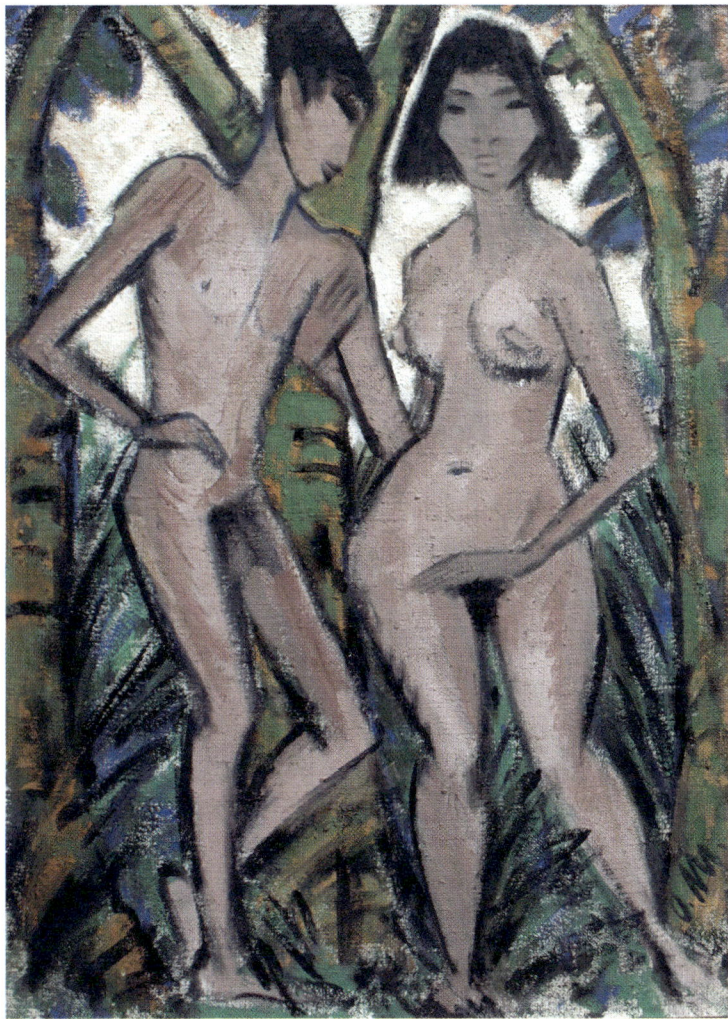

Otto Mueller, *Adam and Eve*, 1918, oil on canvas.

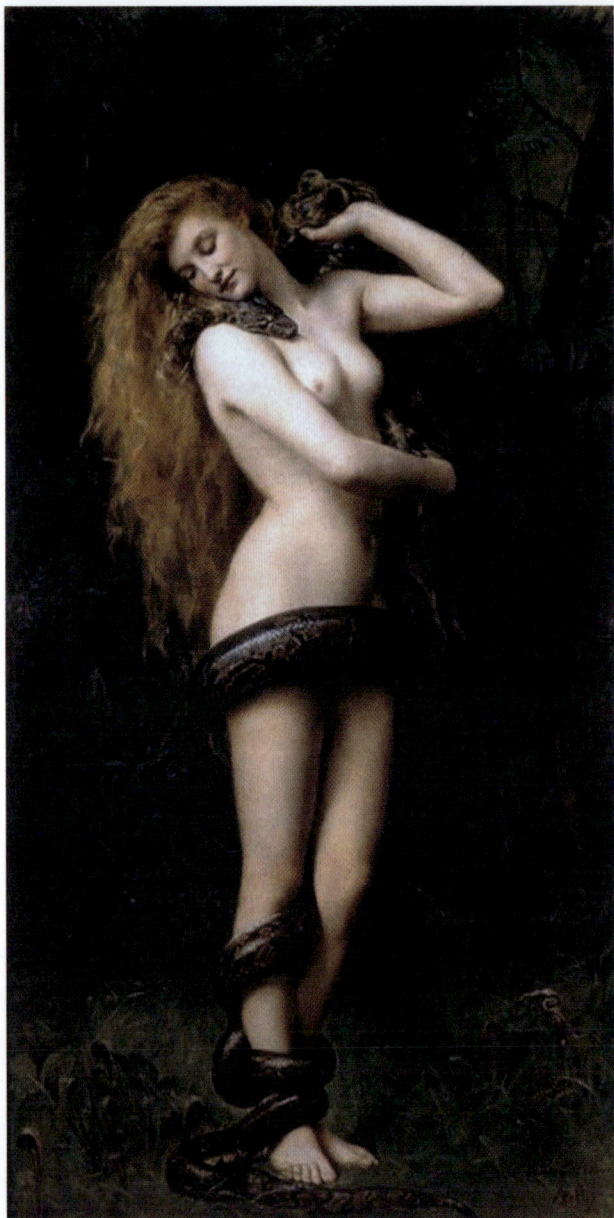

John Collier, *Lilith*, 1892, oil on canvas.

wife, who was created to prevent Adam from coupling with animals. But when Lilith was denied equality with her man, for instance, by demanding to be on top during sexual intercourse, she left him. The Babylonian Talmud describes her as a wild, overly sexed woman. As a folkloric character, Lilith lay with men in their sleep and caused nocturnal emissions and other 'unclean' sexual events. Many scholars trace Lilith and the serpent of Genesis back to the woman and the snake chased from Inanna's Huluppu Tree by Gilgamesh in Sumerian mythology.

Other biblical femme fatale myths have provided us with names that we associate to this day with women who lead men astray with their sexual powers. As noted above, Jezebel, the Phoenician princess, marries the Hebrew king Ahab and uses her feminine powers (charms) to lead him and his people away from the Yahweh religion to the Baal religion of the Canaanites. Under the curse of the prophet Elijah her body after her death was eaten by dogs. The Philistine Delilah seduces the Israelite hero Samson, making him vulnerable to her. While he sleeps, she has the God-given source of his immense strength – his hair – shaved off (she also has him blinded) by her fellow Philistines.

Bathsheba, married to the Hittite Uriah, does not need to actively seduce King David. Her nakedness as he observes her bathing is sufficient. David is so overcome by his desire for Bathsheba that he arranges for the death of her husband in battle and marries her. The union with Bathsheba leads to the birth of Solomon, the future king, but David's actions are obviously shameful and eliciting of Yahweh's wrath. The story of a king disposing of a comrade in war to attain access to the soldier's wife, an act that results finally in the birth of a future king, will be repeated in the legend of King Arthur's conception.

There are cases in the Hebrew Bible in which the charms of femmes fatales are used with positive effect. An example is that of Judith in the book named for her. Judith seduced the Babylonian general Holofernes and then, while he was drunk, she decapitated him, thus saving Israel from defeat in battle.

The femme fatale theme in the Bible reflects a male fear – a sense that the female, through sexual power, can manipulate men and render them vulnerable. In the Book of Proverbs, Solomon warns his son of the power of the adulteress: her lips may 'drip honey' and may be 'smoother than oil' but 'in the end she is as bitter as wormwood, as sharp as a two-edged sword'. This fear, especially as articulated in the Abrahamic cultures, but also in others, has led to the all too general assumption that feminine power must be contained. The means of containment are many. They include the isolation of women from men other than their own family members by way of specified clothing, restrictions of movement, the exclusive control by men of material possessions and land, female circumcision to reduce the possibility of female sexual satisfaction, restrictions around the education of women and their role in politics and religious life, and the emergence of what might be called the cult of virginity, a cult that did not exist, for instance, in Sumer or Egypt.

The Christian addition to the Hebrew Bible (the New Testament) tells of the femme fatale usually thought to be Salome, whose attractiveness to King Herod as she danced before him led the king to promise Salome anything she wanted. What she wanted was the head of John the Baptist and she got it, literally on a platter.

The male fear of female power associated with sex is particularly evident among the early Christian church fathers, who put a great deal of emphasis on the Original Sin of Adam and Eve in the Garden of Eden, generally associating that sin particularly with desire and

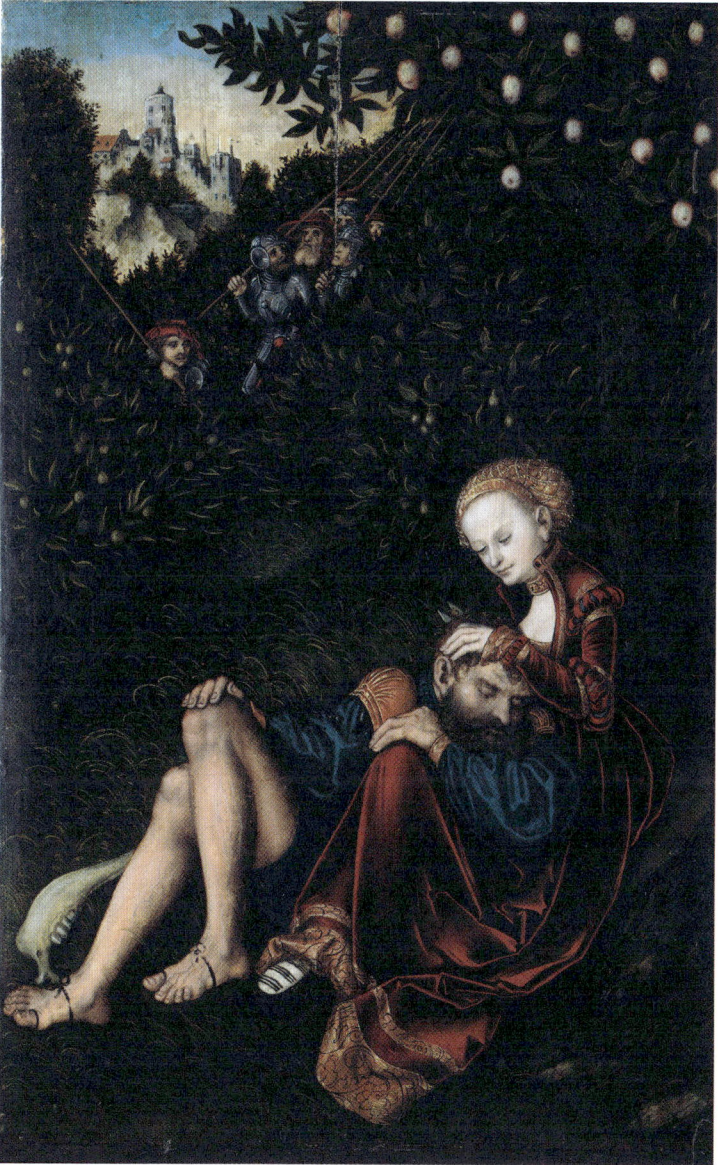

Lucas Cranach the Elder, *Samson and Delilah*, *c.* 1528, oil on beechwood.

sex and women. Tertullian, the North African theologian of the second and third century CE wrote that *all* women, by definition, were femmes fatales. 'Do you [women] not know,' he wrote, 'that you are each an Eve? . . . the "devil's gateway".' And in the fourth century CE St Augustine of Hippo would write, 'What is the difference whether it is a wife or a mother, it is still Eve the temptress that we must be aware of in any woman.'

The Abrahamic traditions manage to circumvent the problem that their heroes must be conceived in sexual activity, the woman's genitals being the only doorway into life, by often making that activity as sexless as possible. The supposedly barren Sarah managed to conceive Isaac with the one-hundred-year-old Abraham when she was ninety. St Elizabeth in the Christian story conceives John the Baptist in a 'barren' womb. St Anne conceives Mary immaculately – that is, somehow without the sexual taint of the Original Sin of Eve.

St Augustine wrote that when Adam disobeyed God, 'the sexual parts of his body were the first to rise up in disobedience', the first sign of Original Sin. Christian mythology, based on the monotheism of its Jewish antecedent, contains an essential paradox which must ultimately involve the penis and the overcoming of its original 'rising up'. The paradox involves God as a male, the doctrine of the Trinity, and the humanity of Jesus. God is seen by Christians – more clearly than is the case for other monotheists, the Jews and the Muslims – as a male figure. He is 'Our Father'. To see God as male is to assume male genitalia. Yet, in monotheism, God can have no sexual consort – no wife, no lover. He does not have sex. The concept of a powerful being who has genitals but chooses not to use them is, to be sure, a positive concept to support ascetic practices such as monasticism and other forms of religious celibacy. But God the 'Father' is inexorably tied in the Christian doctrine of the Trinity to the Son (Jesus) and the Holy Spirit. It is crucial to that doctrine and to Christianity in general that Jesus be a human incarnation of God. To be human he must be born. To be born he must be conceived and must enter the world by way of the female genitals. Christianity solves the obvious problem of sex here by having Jesus conceived in Mary without intercourse through the agency of God in his form as the non-corporeal Holy Spirit. Jesus is then born of Mary who remains a virgin after the birth. The human mind remains fixated in its cultural dreams, however, to established patterns and archetypes. In two late dogmas, Mary is, in effect, deified. In the doctrine of the Immaculate Conception, her own conception is said to have been 'without sin' – that is, without the involvement of what St Augustine would have seen as the sin of sexual desire. In the even later doctrine of the Assumption of the Virgin bodily into Heaven, Mary is enthroned there as Regina Coeli – Queen of Heaven – presumably as God the Father's consort. In mythical terms, the Earth Goddess has been impregnated by God, has given birth to God and has returned to God as his queen. It seems that despite a culture's official dogma, the archetypal pattern will not be denied.

In Islam, too, sex is avoided in connection with Allah. Allah is wifeless, although in pre-Islamic Semitic Arabia he had goddess companions, Al-Lat, Al-Uzza and Manat. Al-Uzza was a fertility goddess, Manat was related to Fate, and Al-Lat, according to Herodotus, was the Arabic form of Aphrodite. If so, she is related to Astarte and the other Semitic goddesses of Mesopotamia and Canaan. Sex within certain rules is not in itself inherently dangerous in Islam if the male, who may have four wives (Muhammad had many more), retains dominance. The female, of course, may not have multiple husbands.

In Judaism sex is not evil. God did command the first couple to be fruitful and multiply, after all. And sex is not always associated in the Hebrew Bible with femmes fatales. There is, for example, the 'Song of Songs', which was appended to the Bible in the second century CE and which probably owes something to the sexual poetry of Mesopotamia concerning Inanna and Dumuzi. The 'Song of Songs' literally revels in sexual love. The beloved in the poem speaks of her lover: 'As the apple tree among the trees of wood, so is my beloved among the sons. I sat down under his shadow with great delight, and his fruit was sweet to my taste.' This is reminiscent of Inanna under the apple tree as she admires her budding sexuality before leaving to meet Enki. The woman in the 'Song of Songs' loses and then finds her lover and, like Inanna, she brings him into her mother's house for love: 'I held him, and would not let him go, until I had brought him into my mother's house, and into the chamber of her that conceived me.' And the lover is not at a loss for words; among many other compliments he says, 'Thy two breasts are like two young roes that are twins, which feed among the lilies.' The woman revels in his words and his love: 'My beloved put his hand by the hole of the door, and my bowels were moved for him. I rose up to open to my beloved; and my hands dropped with myrrh, and my fingers with sweet smelling myrrh, upon the handles of the lock.' Sexual double meanings are obvious here. But both Jews and Christians have traditionally treated the 'Song of Songs' not as a celebration of sex and love between individuals but as allegories of God's love for Israel and for his 'bride', the Church.

Sex is subject to many rules in Judaism. The Book of Leviticus contains a list of sexual acts forbidden by Yahweh, including incest, bestiality and homosexuality. It also outlines in detail the way 'impurity' related to such events as menstruation and other types of bodily fluid emission is to be treated. Islamic law also contains such instructions.

There are many biblical stories of sexual laws being broken in the biblical 'history' of Israel, stories which presumably were thought to stand as negative examples. One of the first of these myths is contained in Genesis 18, in which Abraham is told by three representatives of God that the cities of Sodom and Gomorrah will be destroyed because of their inhabitants' 'grievous' sins. These sins are usually associated with the breaking of God's laws regarding sexuality. We apply the word 'sodomy', from Sodom, to sexual acts that have been forbidden by law at certain times in certain cultures, or to sexual acts other than vaginal intercourse – anal or oral sex, for example – that are forced on an unwilling individual. When Abraham asks God whether Sodom and Gomorrah might be spared because virtuous people surely live there, God agrees that ten righteous people would be a sufficient number to save the cities. So, God sends two angels to visit Sodom, and Abraham's nephew Lot invites them to visit him there. At nightfall, the men of Sodom come to Lot's house and, in effect, accuse Lot of homosexual acts with his visitors, demanding that the men be given to them so that they might 'know' them – that is, have sex with them too. Lot refuses and, making the limited value of women clear, offers the men of Sodom his two virgin daughters instead. The men refuse, and the angels help Lot and his family to escape, as now Sodom and Gomorrah will be destroyed, Lot being the only just man found there. The angels warn the escapees not to look behind them as they leave, but Lot's wife does, and she is turned into a pillar of stone and left behind – the fate of the woman who disobeys (like Orpheus' Eurydice in Greek mythology).

The story does not end there. Living in the wilderness in a cave after the destruction of the evil cities, Lot and his daughters become perpetrators of a primary taboo. The daughters despair of having no sexual partners and thus no progeny, and Genesis 19 records their making their father drunk so that they might sleep with him without his being aware of the incestuous acts. The result is children who are both sons and grandsons to Lot and brothers and sons to the daughters.

A second tragic tale of incest is that of Amnon and Tamar. Amnon was King David's eldest son and heir apparent. He was infatuated by his brother Absalom's sister Tamar (Absalom and Amnon had different mothers, so Tamar was Amnon's half-sister). Having tricked Tamar into coming to him during a pretended illness, he raped her and then abandoned her in disgust. This act led to conflict in David's family; that is, a sexual sin undermined Israel itself. Absalom had his brother murdered in revenge and then led a rebellion against David, even sleeping with his father's concubines as an insult.

Another Tamar, this one in Genesis 38, has a wicked husband who dies. The husband's brother, Onan, according to tradition is told to marry his brother's widow to produce children in the family line. Onan is reluctant to produce children with Tamar for his evil brother, so he practises coitus interruptus and 'spills his seed' on the ground, earning God's wrath for himself. Onan thus gives his name to the term 'onanism', wrongly applied to masturbation rather than to any purposeful 'spilling' of semen outside of the vagina.

A sin mentioned in Leviticus as being particularly evil is that of homosexuality. Yet in the Books of Samuel a story exists that, according to several scholars, would seem to involve David himself in the perceived sin. In 1 Samuel 18 David and Jonathan form a love covenant: 'the soul of Jonathan was knit with the soul of David.' Later, when David hears the news of the death of King Saul and Jonathan, he grieves particularly for Jonathan: 'very pleasant hast thou been unto me: thy love to me was wonderful, passing the love of women.' Does this mean that David and Jonathan were lovers, or is it simply a patriarchal expression of the superior nature of male friendship, males being valued over females? Modern scholarship is divided on the question. The homosexual argument gains strength in Saul's dinner table admonishment of Jonathan for his special friendship with David: 'Thou son of the perverse rebellious *woman*, do not I know that thou hast chosen the son of Jesse [David] to thine own confusion, and unto the confusion of thy mother's nakedness?'

Whether David and Jonathan were lovers or not, their story, like most others in the Bible, reveals a principle of male importance. Ultimately this is an importance based on the penis. In Judaism and Islam, the penis is a central focus, as established in God's ordering Abraham and his people to undergo the removal of the foreskin as a sign of the covenant with the divine. Although female circumcision is prevalent in some Islamic societies, male circumcision is a universal Jewish and Islamic ritual and is in itself by definition inherently phallocentric, making the circumcised penis the defining symbol of membership in the larger community – the 'chosen people' and the Ummah.

For Christians, circumcision has never been a requirement, primarily because the apostle Paul – formerly the Jewish zealot Saul – associated circumcision with Judaism and wished to emphasize that the new religion, of which he was the primary proponent, was fully open to Gentiles, the uncircumcised. Paul, however, contributed to the concept of the secondary nature of women, as opposed to men, in society and particularly in the practice of the new religion. In his first letter to the Christian church in Corinth, he makes his position clear: during worship women must cover their heads while men must leave their heads uncovered (could the 'uncovered' head be an unconscious reference to circumcision on Paul's part – a metaphorical circumcision for Gentiles?) 'because a man is the image of God, whereas a woman reflects the glory of man.' And later:

> Let your women keep silence in the churches: for it is not
> permitted unto them to speak; but they are commanded
> to be under obedience, as also saith the law.
> And if they will learn anything, let them ask their husbands
> at home: for it is a shame for women to speak in church
> (1 Corinthians 14:34–5)

The combination of Eve's sexual 'sin' and Paul's commands rooted in traditional Judaism has kept women in a secondary position in much of Christianity to this day, limiting their liturgical role, for instance, in the most ancient and largest of the Christian denominations, Roman Catholicism.

If Semitic mythology in Mesopotamia indicates a change in attitudes towards sexuality, the Semitic mythologies of the Canaanites and Israelites perpetuated the conflict that led to that change. For Canaanites, sex, whether as experienced by mythological figures or as celebrated in rituals, was clearly associated with the fertility of the land, with climate and successful agriculture. Tempting as this understanding was to the agriculturalist Hebrews who came to Canaan, it was in direct conflict with their monotheism. Yahweh was a god without a mate, a jealous god who ruled alone, without the sexual appetite of the gods of the cultures that surrounded him. His prophets knew that sex was a powerful instinct which could lead people away from their sacred covenant. Sex could be controlled and directed appropriately by laws that could curtail and redirect the drives represented by the likes of Eve and the biblical femmes fatales, the drives represented so powerfully by El and Baal and by the gods of the neighbouring Greeks.

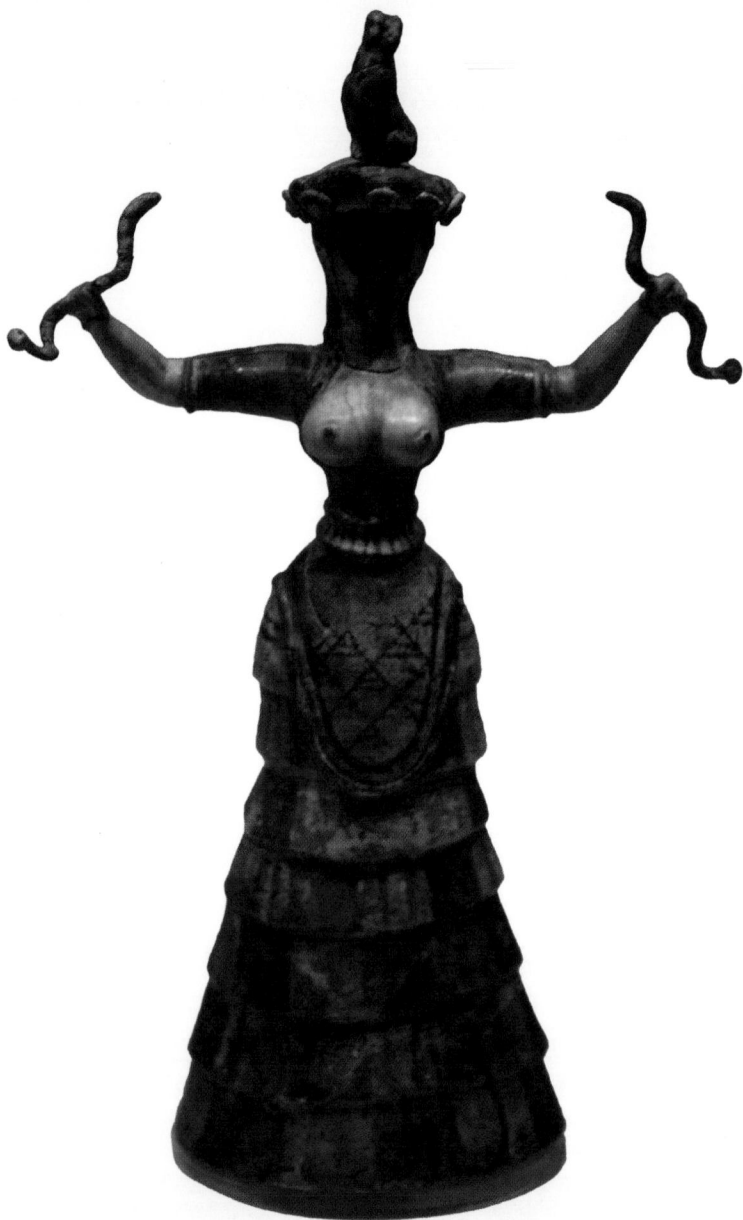

Minoan snake goddess, Crete, *c.* 1600 BCE, quartz faience.

Four

Greece and Rome

WHILE THE SUMERIANS and Egyptians were emerging as great cultures, and the Hebrews had not yet entered Canaan, an early form of what we now think of as the ancient Greek civilization was developing on the island of Crete. The people of Crete have long been called Minoans, after their mythical King Minos, who, according to later Greeks, was the son of Europa, a maiden Zeus forcibly abducted – that is, raped. Recent studies indicate that the Minoans were, indeed, children of Europe, if Europa is a symbol of the European continent. In fact, many scholars have long believed that the Minoans descended from Anatolian tribes who migrated to Europe in the seventh millennium BCE and may have spoken a language that was, in effect, the ancestor of Greek and other Indo-European languages. High Minoan culture thrived from about 2700 BCE (some say earlier) until it was overthrown by Mycenaean Greeks in about 1450 BCE.

The Minoans had writing systems beginning in about 2000 BCE. But their mythology must be considered prehistoric since the writing systems – Minoan hieroglyphic and so-called Linear A – have yet to be deciphered. Until Minoan writing is deciphered, Minoan mythology can only be known by way of archaeological ruins and works of art.

Apparently, the name Minos was applied to all Cretan kings, also beginning in about 2000 BCE. It has been suggested by Robert Graves and others that Minos means 'Moon Man' and that a tradition is likely to have existed in which a ritual marriage and sexual union took place between the priest-king and a representative of a Great Goddess in her form as moon deity. If so, such marriages might have resembled those in Mesopotamia and Canaan. Certainly, goddesses – perhaps various embodiments of a single Great Goddess – are prevalent in Cretan art. The best known of these embodiments is the 'snake goddess', depicted holding up snakes in each hand. The snake, probably because it sheds and replaces its old skin annually, is commonly associated with fertility and thus with goddesses who, as females, embody birth-giving fertility.

The Minoan snake goddess has been associated with the Phoenician goddess Astarte, another goddess of fertility. This association is supported by the myth of Zeus' rape of Europa since, according to the story, Europa was a Phoenician princess, and Zeus carried her off to Crete.

The snake goddess, depicted in frescoes and figurines in Cretan cave sanctuaries and ruins, is clearly a sexual being of great power. Her breasts are bare and exaggerated and her pubic area is often highlighted with a triangular form in a tradition extending back to the Palaeolithic 'Venuses'. Sometimes the goddess is shown in fields accompanied by adoring male dancers or animals. A common companion is a youth the mainland Greeks believed was the boy Zeus or the boy Dionysos.

As in other ancient myths of the Great Goddess – the Çatal Hüyük Venus, Inanna/Ishtar or Anat, for example – the bull is a significant element and always a sexual one, as in the myth in which Zeus takes the form of a bull to abduct Europa. There are several myths, in addition to the Europa story, told and written in mainland Greece but based on Minoan themes. The myth of Daedalus and Icarus is an example. Some scholars believe that these myths were, in fact, originally Minoan, and that they may have been imported into mainland Greece from Crete by the Mycenaeans. The most erotic of the Crete-based myths is that of Queen Pasiphae, the Bull of Poseidon, and the Minotaur.

According to the myth, when Minos first proclaimed himself King of Crete he made the common mistake of prideful heroes by boasting that he was favoured by the gods, who would always answer his prayers. Minos then erected an altar to Poseidon at which he requested that he be sent a bull which he would then sacrifice to the gods. Immediately, Minos' boast seemed to be justified as a great white bull emerged from the realm of the sea god. But Minos so admired the bull that he broke his promise, placed it in his own herds and chose another – by definition, inferior – bull for the ritual sacrifice.

The gods do not reward duplicity, and Poseidon took historic revenge. Divine retribution against humans often takes the form of forbidden sexuality, as other Greek myths make particularly clear. In this case the god Poseidon chooses bestiality. He causes Minos' wife, Pasiphae, to lust after the bull. The queen becomes so desperate that she enlists Daedalus, the master craftsman in the employ of the court, to help her 'have her way' with the bull. Daedalus has for some time made life-like dolls for the Cretan royal family and now he uses his expertise to create a hollow wooden cow in which Pasiphae can arrange herself in such a way as to make her vagina available to the deceived bull.

The bull soon arrives and gives Pasiphae the pleasure for which she has yearned.

In the world of mytho-logic, bestiality, like other 'sinful' sexual unions, is exposed as such in the progeny resulting from the given act. Inappropriate sex has its own logical reward, and Pasiphae gives birth to the part-bull, part-human monster, the Minotaur, the shameful beast for which Daedalus is now hired to make a lair, the Labyrinth (which was not a labyrinth but a maze) in which to hide the queen's sin from the world.

Greek myths are all parts of a continuing larger story, and from the Pasiphae myth we move in Greek mythology into the story of

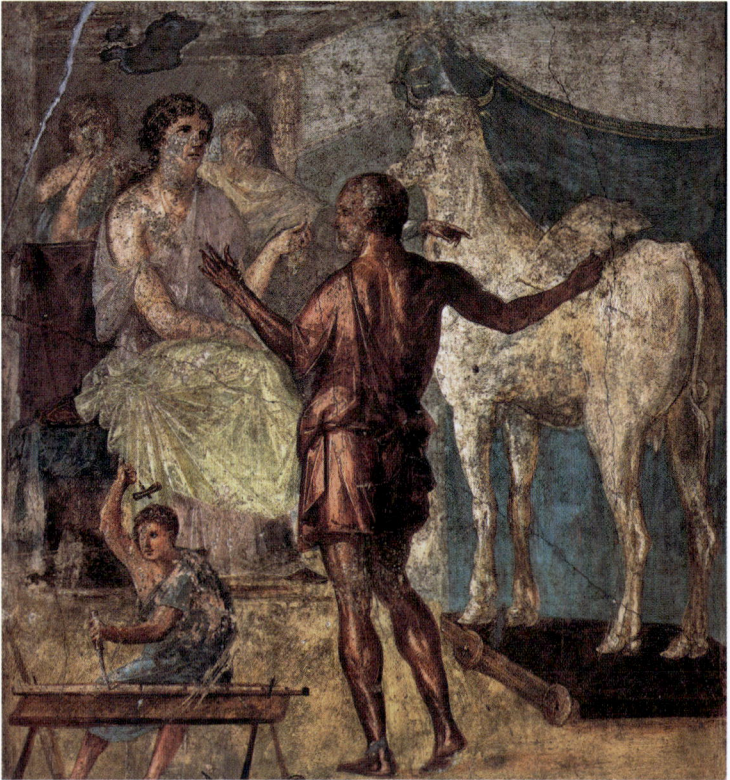

Pasiphae with Daedalus and the false cow, Graeco-Roman fresco, Pompeii, 1st century CE.

Theseus, who would slay the Minotaur and escape Crete with the help of his lover, the Cretan princess Ariadne, who he would callously abandon on the island of Naxos on his way home to Athens.

The story of Pasiphae may well be a mainland Greek myth told by the Mycenaeans to belittle their rivals, the Minoans. Certainly, the myth seems to be more pornographic than religious, and pornographic mythology was present in abundance in Greece in written form, on vases, statuary and other art forms, often used as a method of satire or comedy. As for the story of the defeat of the Minotaur by Theseus, it can be traced to the mainland Mycenaeans and can serve as a metaphor for the Mycenaean conquest of Crete.

The Mycenaeans thrived in mainland Greece from about 1650 BCE until their mysterious collapse in about 1200 BCE. These were the people we know most colourfully by way of the mythology found in Homer's *Iliad* and *Odyssey*, and in the much later works of the famous Greek playwrights Aeschylus, Sophocles and Euripides. It is a mythology centred on the Trojan War and its aftermath: the mythology of Menelaus, Helen, Agamemnon, Clytemnestra, Odysseus and Penelope. If the Trojan War took place, it would likely have been a struggle for control of the Dardanelles in about 1200 BCE, roughly coinciding with the end of the Mycenaean civilization.

By 1450 BCE, at about the time of their invasion and defeat of Crete, the Mycenaeans had developed a syllabic script for their Indo-European language, a form of Greek. The Greek alphabet would only come into being several centuries later. The early Mycenaean script is known as Linear B. It was discovered by Sir Arthur Evans in Crete early in the twentieth century and deciphered by Michael Ventris and John Chadwick in the 1950s. Linear B was a somewhat awkward application of the Mycenaean language to the Minoan Linear A system. In its early form, it was useful for inventories and other lists but not for literary purposes. Linear B lists do, however, contain essential elements of the Olympian mythology that we most commonly associate with the ancient Greeks. Zeus (Diwe) is present, as is Hera (Era). Other Olympians present are Poseidon (Posedaone), Athena (Atana Potinija), Apollo (Pajawone), Artemis (Atemito), Hermes (Emaa), Ares (Are), Hephaistos (Apaitoji), Dionysos (Diwonusojo) and Demeter (Da-mater, the Earth Mother). Aphrodite is missing but will emerge later in post-Mycenaean Greece by way of Cyprus from Phoenicia, probably a version of the collective Canaanite/Mesopotamian love goddess.

Other than a list of deities, there is little that Linear B can tell us about Mycenaean mythology. Martin Nilsson in his classic *The Mycenaean Origin of Greek Mythology* (1932) sees Mycenaean civilization, centred around a conquest-oriented warrior aristocracy, as a ripe source for heroic tales and myths that would have been passed along orally by minstrels and other storytellers until they were given more specific form by compilers and poets such as Homer and Hesiod sometime between 850 and 700 BCE, and much later, in the fifth century BCE, by the Athenian playwrights. These dates are open to question, but in about 1200 BCE Mycenaean civilization gave way to what is called the Greek Dark Ages, perhaps initiated by natural causes, perhaps, as some claim, by an invasion of other Indo-Europeans from the north, the Dorians. The era known as the Archaic Period (800–480 BCE), the period of Homer and Hesiod, was one of cultural awakening that would lead to the classical period in which the myths and legends reaching all the way back to the Minoans would finally take written form, giving us what we now know as 'Greek mythology', the mythology that, with later elaboration by the Roman poets Virgil and Ovid, and along with the stories of the Bible, has most influenced the Western world.

Greek mythology is nothing if not sexual, but the sex in these myths is not the sacred sex of Inanna's hymns or the voluptuous loving sex of the 'Song of Songs'. With few exceptions, it is violent, abusive, cruel, misogynistic and nearly always outside the boundaries of accepted human behaviour. At the same time, it is sex based firmly in the patriarchal traditions of the hierarchical Indo-European social system. The myths in which humans and gods connect, for instance, convey a pessimistic sense of the helplessness the Greeks must have felt in relation to their gods. The females ravished by Zeus and other gods are representative of the position of all people subject to families of arbitrary and selfish beings. The myths clearly reflect the historical and sociological reality of the inferior status of women in Greek society.

In aristocratic warrior and male-dominated Mycenae, women had a certain amount of freedom and sometimes even power, but ultimately they too existed for the convenience of men. Later, in 'democratic' Athens, women were not voting citizens and were, in effect, owned by their fathers and husbands. Ancient Greek women were expected to be virgins until they were married, usually by their early teens, often to much older men. The concept of female consent was as irrelevant as the concept of human free will in relation to the gods.

The chronology of the Greek mythological story as we know it begins with the creation and establishment of deities who would eventually give way to the new Olympian gods in a war in Heaven. Hesiod tells the tale in his *Theogony*, likely synthesizing material passed down orally from Crete and Mycenae and possibly from other Near Eastern civilizations such as those of Mesopotamia and Canaan and the Hurrians and Hittites of Anatolia. Sex plays a significant role in the Greek creation story.

In the beginning, Hesiod tells us, there was only the void (Chaos), out of which emerged Gaia (Mother Earth) and Eros (uncontrollable Desire). Gaia's first creation was Ouranos (Sky), who, as in so many other creation myths, immediately 'covered' the creatrix in an endless act of intercourse resulting in a huge litter of monsters and terrifying gods, including the Cyclops and the Titans, among whom were Prometheus, Atlas, the Earth Goddess Rhae and her eventual husband Kronos (Time).

As in Sumer (An and Ki), Egypt (Geb and Nut) and many other cultures, this union of Sky and Earth was suffocating, more so in this case because Ouranos had no use for his offspring, forcing them back into their mother until, in despair, she made a sickle and urged her children to use it to remove their father from her. Kronos, living out in advance an aspect of the twentieth-century Freudian myth, gladly accepted the mission, using the sickle to castrate his father, thus separating the primal parents and leaving room between them for further creation. In castrating his father and thus becoming king of the gods, Kronos keeps company with other castrators of Near Eastern mythology. In Egypt Horus castrates Set and becomes king. In the Hurrian/Hittite cultures of Anatolia (Asian Turkey), the god Kumbari takes power by biting off the testicles of his father Anu (Sky).

Hesiod relates how Kronos flung his father's testicles into the sea, where 'foam' (semen) from them produced the goddess of love and sexuality, Aphrodite, who was always accompanied by her son Eros, a new version of the original Eros (Desire). Aphrodite was not given the status of her Mesopotamian, Egyptian and Canaanite mythological sisters. She was the goddess of irrational passion in the later Olympian pantheon, the femme fatale par excellence.

Meanwhile, blood from the castration of Ouranos fell on Gaia, causing her to conceive and give birth to various giants and, most

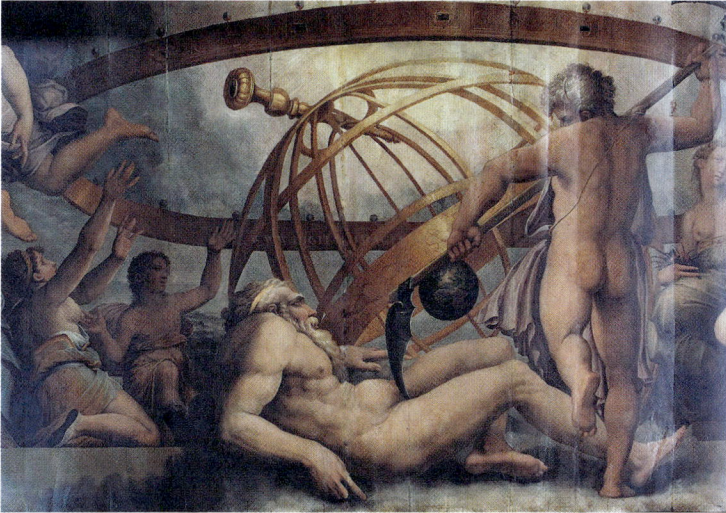

Giorgio Vasari, *Kronos Castrates Ouranos* (The Mutilation of Uranus by Saturn), *c.* 1550, fresco.

importantly, to the dreaded Erinyes, the goddesses of vengeance, who would give unforgiving pain to the Greeks until their taming much later by the more rational Olympians, Apollo and Athena, at which time they were renamed the Eumenides (The Kindly Ones).

With the defeat of Ouranos, Gaia loses her place of dominance in Heaven. Robert Graves sees this mythological fact as a metaphor for the demise of an ancient matriarchal culture. There is evidence, in fact, that Gaia once reigned as the primary deity at the great oracular shrine of Delphi, the omphalos or navel of Gaia (Earth) herself. Later the Olympian god Apollo would arrive to usurp her role, a usurpation signified by his killing of the goddess's great python protector.

After separating his parents and becoming king of Heaven (and later the well-known and much feared Father Time wielding his sickle) Kronos takes his sister Rhae as a wife, in keeping with the tradition of incest among gods. As new versions of Earth and Sky, Kronos and Rhae continue the mating process of their parents. But having replaced his abusive father, Kronos worries that the same fate might await him, so he systematically swallows his children as they are born. The myth refigures what psychology tells us today: child abuse breeds more child abuse.

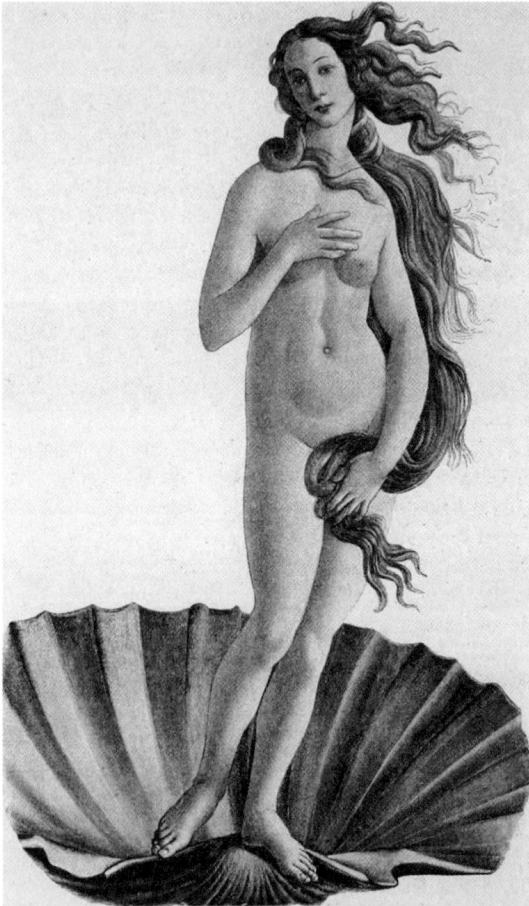

Sandro Botticelli, *The Birth of Venus*,
c. 1483, tempera on canvas.

These children are the first generation of the Olympian gods, Hestia, Demeter, Hera, Hades and Poseidon. Hermes, Ares, Apollo, Athene, Hephaistos, Dionysos and Aphrodite will be incorporated into the family later. Like her mother, Rhae resents the brutality of her mate and acts against him. She substitutes a rock for her sixth born, the baby Zeus, sending the hidden child to Crete to be nursed there by his grandmother Gaia. Irritated by the swallowed rock, Kronos vomits up his first five children, whom Zeus will later lead in a war against their father and the Titans. After victory Zeus becomes king of Heaven, situating his throne on Mount Olympus, establishing himself firmly as leader of the gods known collectively as the Olympians. Zeus' supplanting of the old gods resembles Marduk's rise in Babylon and Baal's in Canaan.

Hesiod, Homer and later myth-makers tell many stories of the sexual activities of Zeus and his Olympian family. There is sex between gods, between gods and lesser divine beings – nymphs are popular mates – and between immortals and humans. It can be argued that sexual activity is a primary defining factor of what is, after all, the official ancient Greek religion. When we think of the Greek head god, Zeus, for instance, we think of thunderbolts and arbitrary power, but we also think of his philandering.

Several of Zeus' conquests involve rape and bestiality. As a bull, he abducts the princess Europa. In a much-depicted act, he takes the form of a swan to rape Leda, Queen of Lacedaemon (Sparta). In some versions of the Leda myth Leda lays two eggs, which hatch, providing the world with the twins Castor and Polydeuces (Pollux) and, more tragically, Helen and Clytemnestra, two femmes fatales who would play major parts in the Trojan War and its aftermath. The bestiality in the Zeus myths and the Pasiphae myth is not an indication that bestiality was a popular Greek pastime, however. Both

Greeks and Romans associated the practice with satyrs and especially with the wild god Pan.

Zeus did not always take animal guises to have his way with mortal women. He became a shower of gold in order to impregnate Danae, princess of Argos. The resulting progeny was the hero Perseus, who killed Medusa.

The god king was not only interested in women. At one point, he lusted after the beautiful semi-divine boy Ganymede. Homosexuality as a negative concept was apparently irrelevant to Zeus. He became an eagle and carried the boy off to Mount Olympus to be his cup bearer.

It should be said that events such as these in Greek mythology likely were intended to be funny on one hand and indicative of heavenly arbitrariness on the other. They were not, for instance, metaphors for a deeper spiritual union between humanity and the divine. In fact, spirituality seems to have had only a small place in

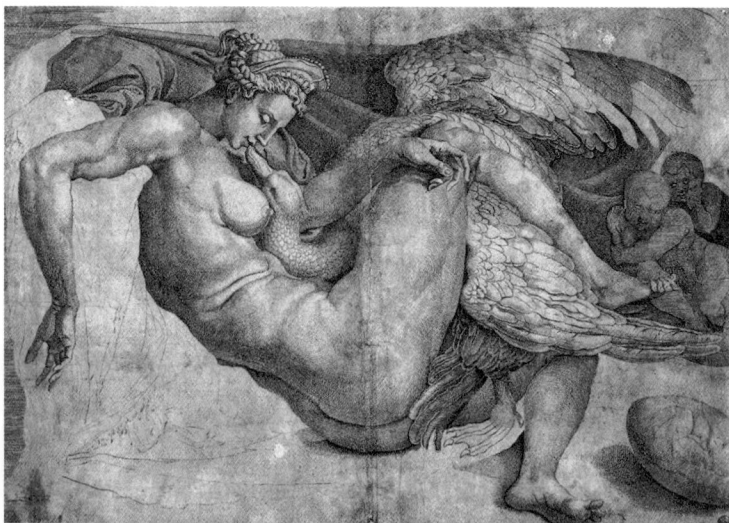

Cornelis Bos, *Leda and the Swan*, c. 1550, engraving.

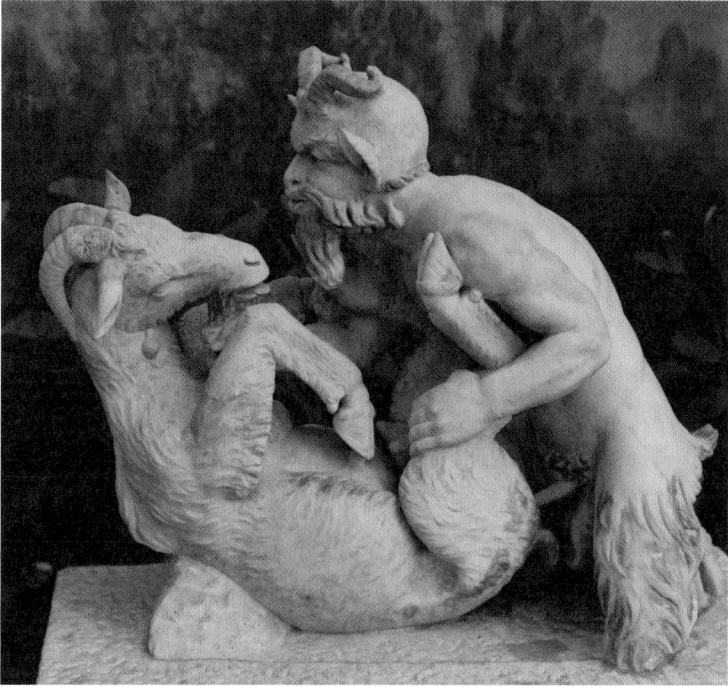

Statue of Pan with a goat, Herculaneum, 1st century CE.

Greek mythology. It is present by implication at least in the narratives about certain pederastic homosexual relationships.

Much has been written about the existence of pederasty in ancient Greece. Its acceptable form, possibly originating in Minoan Crete, involved a relationship between a young man (*erastes* or *philetor*) and a younger adolescent boy (*eremos* or *kleinos*), with the consent of the boy's family. Sometimes the relationship began with a ritual kidnapping, as in the case of Zeus and Ganymede. The man became, in effect, a military, athletic and citizenship trainer of the boy. Sex is generally assumed to have been expected in the relationship, especially given the unavailability of women other than prostitutes and the commonplace of nudity among males in gymnasiums and athletic fields. Sex

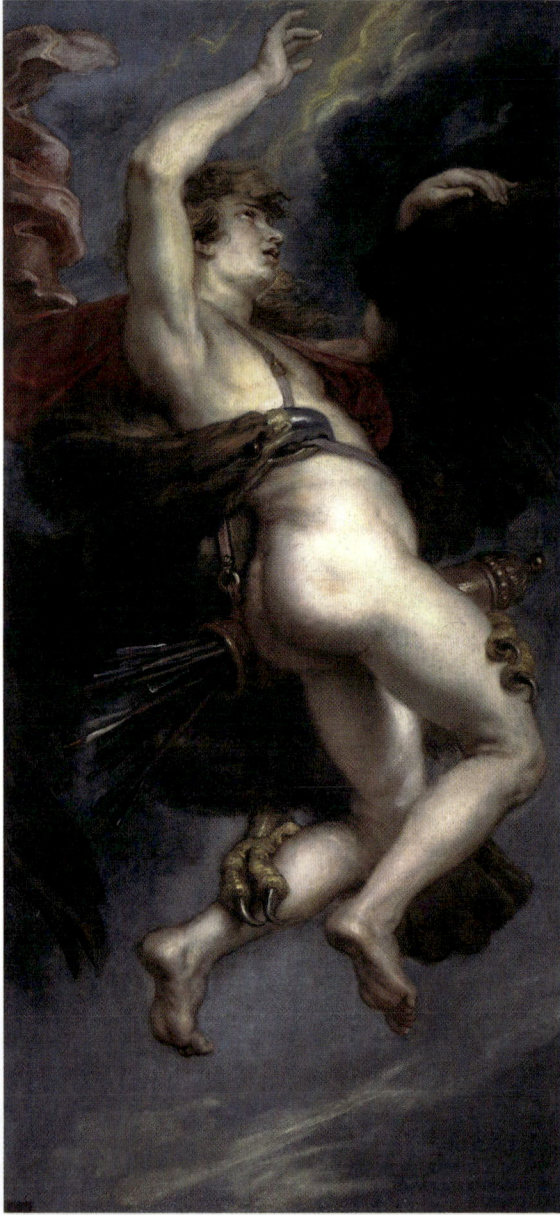

Peter Paul Rubens, *The Rape of Ganymede*, 1636–8, oil on canvas.

between the man and boy would have been considered proper if the active role was the man's.

Several popular myths convey a sense of positive pederasty in Greece, myths in which the relationships in question approach the level of spiritual love between individuals. The most famous of these myths is the one about the god Apollo and his constant companion and apparent lover, the beautiful boy Hyacinth. One day Apollo and the boy were practising discus throwing, athletics being a normal part of the kind of relationship they represented. A jealous rival for Hyacinth's love was the West Wind, Zephyr, who caused one of Apollo's discuses to hit Hyacinth in the head, ending his life. Grief-stricken, Apollo caused Hyacinth's spilled blood to result in the springing to life of the Hyacinth flower.

Other such myths involve the great hero Herakles, the epitome of powerful manliness. Herakles had boy lovers, including his own nephew Iolaus and the beautiful Hylas, who left him to live with nymphs, and sent the hero into a period of deep despair.

A relationship often used to illustrate male homosexuality in Greece is that between Achilles and his beloved companion Patroclos in Homer's *Iliad*. Certainly, the relationship is closer than other male relationships depicted in the epic. The difficulties of interpretation here resemble those relating to the Jonathan and David relationship in the Bible. Was the deep love between the heroes an example of physical love or was it, as seems more likely, another example of the spiritual value attributed in highly patriarchal societies to male relationships, whether sexual or not?

As in other ancient cultures there is a comic and pornographic element in the treatment of homosexuality in Greek culture, especially if same sex acts fell outside of the boundaries of the almost spiritual unions described above. Certain vase paintings, for instance,

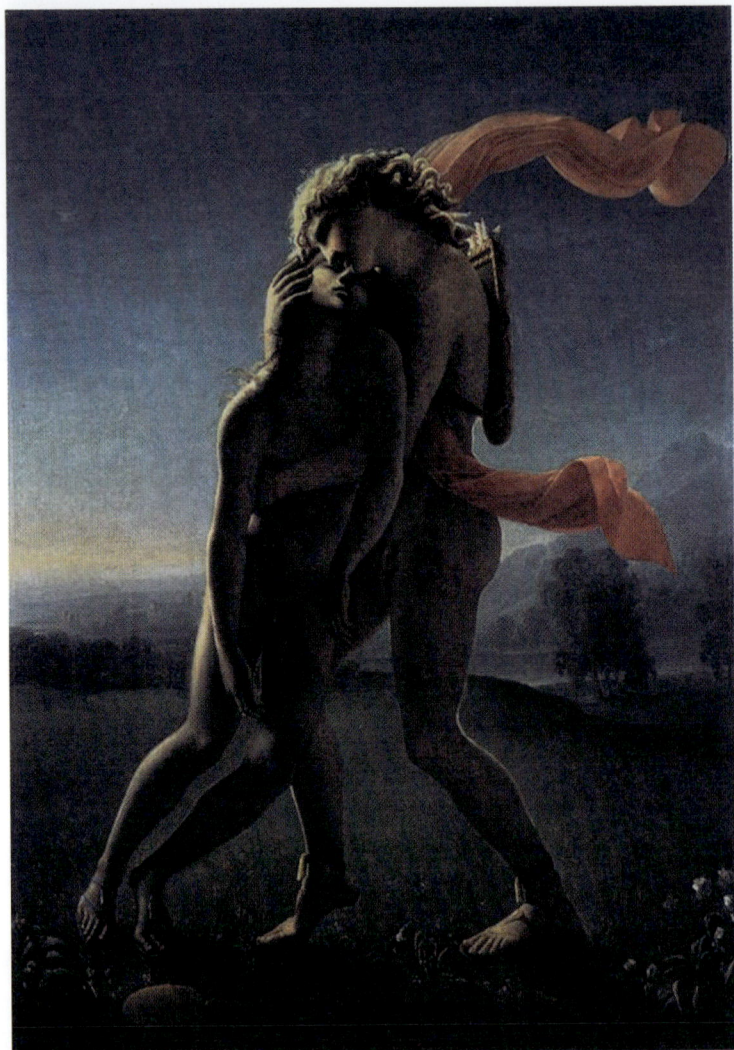

Jean Broc, *The Death of Hyacinth*, 1801, oil on canvas.

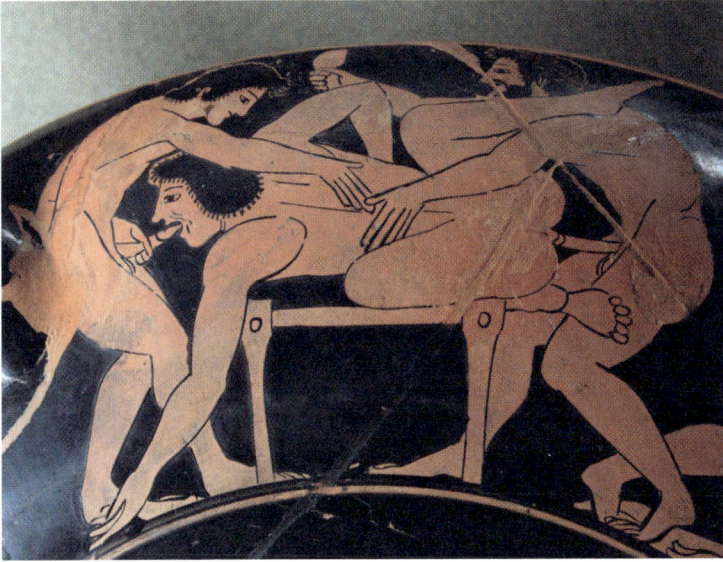

A homosexual scene on an Attic Greek kylix (wine-drinking bowl), *c.* 510 BCE.

portray a view of homosexuality which is at once orgiastic, comic and pornographic.

A comparison of sex as depicted in the mythology of the Bible with sex as depicted in Greek mythology reveals a marked difference between the points of view of the two mythologies that have been so influential on 'Western' culture. For the compilers of the Bible there was only one God, and he had no sexual activity unless we count his impregnation of Mary in the New Testament, an impregnation that was accomplished asexually without the loss of the maiden's virginity. Sex in the Bible, then, involves only humans with each other, and in most cases this sex can be seen to serve as a precaution against femmes fatales and / or the breaking of established religious rules. The emphasis on sexuality in the Bible is a 'Thou shalt not' emphasis. Sex in Greek mythology, on the other hand, involves many gods and other non-humans, so there is more than ample opportunity for Olympian sex outside of the human realm. The sex that does take place between the gods and humans is clearly not intended to teach morality or ethics or to emphasize religious standards. Olympian sex, as noted earlier, is almost always outside of the boundaries of accepted *human* behaviour. It reflects a sense among the Greeks that the gods, rather than standing as symbols of morality, represent our worst tendencies towards misogyny and self-serving. Regarding Olympian sex, it is useful to consider the theologian and philosopher Martin Buber's differentiation between I–it and I–thou. In an I–it relationship the individual sees the object of desire as an 'it' who has nothing to do with spirituality or the inner self. In the I–thou relationship two individuals relate to each other without objectification, as two loving beings. The Greek gods, with rare exceptions, relate sexually to each other and especially to humans in the I–it context. In this they are players in a continuing human predilection for pornography. Pornography is essentially male fantasy involving either a strangely willing or a raped victim and a list of such possibilities as incest, bestiality, the possession of young women by older men, and the tricking of disrespected women into activities that have everything to do with male pleasure and nothing to do with what we think of as love or spirituality or the development of viable romantic relationships.

The extended Olympian family is a family made for I–it erotic soap opera. At the head of the family is the great philanderer Zeus, who has infinite power and can take what he wants. His wife Hera is a stereotypically nagging wife, who spends much of her time plotting revenge against her husband's sexual victims. One such victim, for example, is poor Io, whom Zeus turns into a cow to disguise her from Hera. Hera discovers the deception and has a gadfly chase the cow across the world, torturing her constantly with its stings (thus the Ionian Sea and the Bosporus – 'Cow's ford'). In another example, when Hera discovers that the mortal woman Alcmene is pregnant by Zeus she tries unsuccessfully to have the goddess of childbirth prevent the birth, essentially by crossing the young woman's legs. The child in question was later named Herakles ('Hera's Glory') because Athene tricked Hera into nursing him.

Hera did occasionally enjoy sexual relations with her husband, but usually only to achieve ulterior goals. In the *Iliad* Homer describes how Hera uses some Aphrodite love charms to attract the great philanderer to her bed. Then, later, while he sleeps off his carnal activities, she can manipulate things to her liking in the Trojan War.

Zeus' highly entitled older brothers, Hades and Poseidon, are, among other things, ruthless sexual predators. One of Hades' heinous acts is the subject of one of the most popular of Greek myths. Perhaps to rid Olympus of serious rivals, Zeus sent Hades to Hades to be king there, and Poseidon to the sea to be head god there. Meanwhile, he had an affair with his older sister Demeter, to whom he assigned the fertility of earth itself as Earth Mother. The result of this liaison was the beautiful Persephone. While wandering among the flowers of a field one day the maiden's uncle, Hades, sprang from the underworld and abducted her. In despair at the loss of her daughter, Demeter neglected the earth, which became barren until Zeus, as Persephone's father, convinced Hades to release the girl. The release could be accomplished, however, only if Persephone had not eaten food of the underworld. Persephone had, in fact, eaten seeds of pomegranate there. The consuming of the underworld food was very likely a metaphor for the loss of virginity, making her Hades' queen and making it impossible for her to spend more than half of the year away from her husband. This arrangement caused alternations in Demeter's moods and resulted in the seasons.

Poseidon was as bad as Zeus and Hades. Like Zeus he had sexual relations with his sister, and in this case rape was the method. When he accosted her Demeter turned herself into a mare to avoid his advances. But the god turned himself into a stallion and raped the mare. According to the Roman poet Ovid, Poseidon also raped a priestess of Athene, who would be punished for being raped by being turned into the monstrous Medusa. The blaming of women for being raped is a fact that has long been an aspect of human society.

Some of the younger members of the Olympian family – the off-spring of the original Olympians – absorbed the licentious ways of their parents and uncles. Aphrodite, born of the 'foam' of Ouranos, was eventually adopted by Zeus as his daughter. Known for her unbridled love of sex, Aphrodite was vain and was responsible for much mischief both on Olympus and in the human world. One indirect result of her sexual charms was the Trojan War. Angry at not having been invited to a wedding attended by the other gods, Eris, the Goddess of Discord, threw a golden apple into the party. The apple was to belong to the 'fairest one'. Hera, Athene and Aphrodite all claimed the prize and Paris, a Trojan prince, was chosen as the judge, Zeus wisely avoiding what could only be a dangerous decision in a family such as his. The goddesses stripped and Paris chose Aphrodite after she promised him the most beautiful human woman as a prize. This was Helen, the wife of King Menelaus of Sparta. To gain access to Helen, Paris had to take her by force from Menelaus' court (some say she fell in love with Paris and went willingly). In any case, the abduction triggered the Mycenaean attack on Troy. Aphrodite's charms, then, led to the destruction of a civilization.

Aphrodite had many affairs. With her stepbrother Dionysos, she produced a son Priapus, whose constant erection reflected her powers (we take the adjective *priapic*, referring to male sexual excitement, from this god). With her stepbrother Hermes, whom, with the help of her adopted father Zeus, she seduced and had a brief affair with, she eventually gave birth to Hermaphroditus, a beautiful combination of the two gods, male and female. This combination, for Plato, was the original androgynous wholeness of a golden age before humans became split into male and female. In this context, the longing of men and women for each other might be a longing to return to the original androgyny, a positive expression of what Shakespeare's Iago would refer to as 'the beast with two backs'.

Hermes himself had a phallocentric aspect in that *herms*, stone pillars topped by his head, frequently sported erect phalli. Ubiquitous in ancient Greece, *herms* were placed in front of homes to ward off

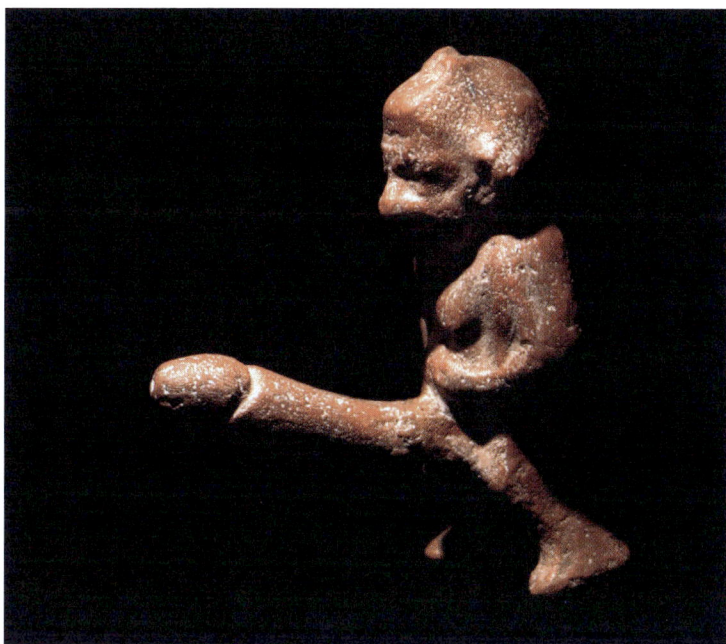

Priapos, Greek terracotta statue, 2nd century CE.

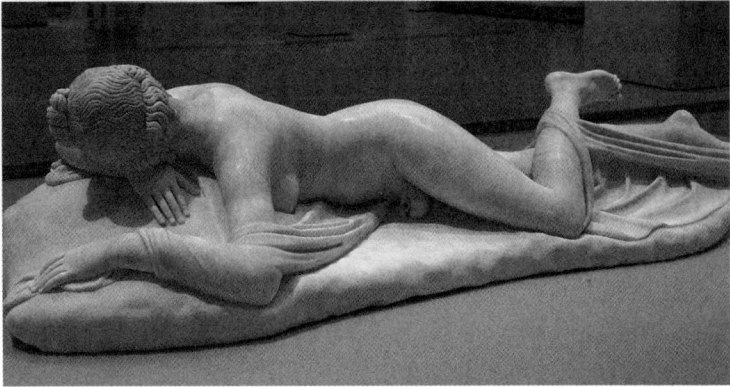

Sleeping Hermaphroditus, attributed to Polycles, 130–50 CE.

evil. It is possible that the erect phallus celebrated the power of the god to penetrate the underworld.

Aphrodite had a husband, the lame blacksmith god Hephaestus, whom she had been forced by Zeus to marry and with whom she was bored. Her most famous affair, with her strong and handsome stepbrother Ares, god of war, was exposed by Hephaestus. Jealous of the affair, he devised a net which he used to capture the lovers *in flagrante delecto* for all the family to see and ridicule.

Two of Aphrodite's sisters, Athene and Artemis, have very different approaches to sex. They are the divine feminists, using their virginity to celebrate their strength as women with no need of men. There is one myth that suggests the possibility of lesbian love on the part of Artemis. Zeus lusted after the nymph Callisto and disguised himself as Artemis to achieve his goal. That the girl, devoted to Artemis, willingly participated at first in the embrace of the partner she believes is the goddess suggests that this might not have been the first such contact between the two. Whatever her view of lesbian sex, Artemis had a dislike of men in a sexual context. When poor Actaeon was hunting one day in the woods, he inadvertently came upon Artemis (in Ovid's version she has the Roman name, Diana) bathing in a pond. Furious at having been seen naked, Artemis turns the young man into a stag, causing his dogs to turn against him, tearing him to pieces.

 The Olympian Greek Artemis takes a very different form from her mythological ancestor in Anatolia, the so-called Artemis of Ephesus, who sported many breasts (or gourds) and was a fertility goddess more related to the Phrygian Mother Goddess Cybele than to the canonical Artemis of the Greek religion.

 Athene was Zeus' favourite daughter, literally born from his head after he swallowed her mother, Metis. Athene was a warrior – a somewhat masculinized goddess – the opposite of her sister Aphrodite, but she did have favourites among men, especially the mortal heroes Odysseus, Perseus and Herakles. She sometimes seems almost to be flirting with Odysseus as she guides him home after the Trojan War. She helps Perseus in his quest to kill Medusa, and she supports Herakles in the accomplishment of his famous twelve labours. But sex was not an activity that interested Athene. Like Artemis, she was devoted to virginity.

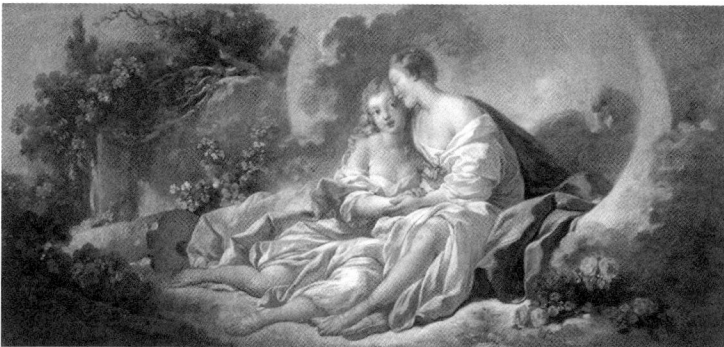

Jean-Honoré Fragonard, *Jupiter Disguised as Diana Makes Love to Callisto*, 1755, oil on canvas.

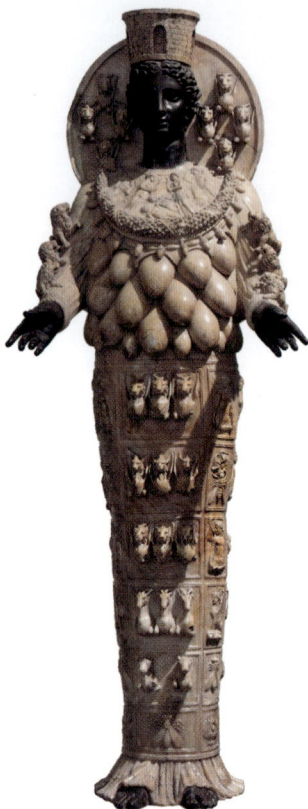

Artemis of Ephesus, Roman statue, 2nd century CE.

Athene was not the only one of Zeus' children to be born of his body. Dionysos, too, was Zeus-born. He was an outsider god, not even usually included in the lists of the twelve Olympians, primarily because, unlike anyone else in the immediate family, he was conceived by a mortal woman. His mother was Semele, the daughter of King Cadmus of Thebes. Zeus had made love to the princess without revealing his real self. Hera discovered the relationship and, disguised as a friendly crone, convinced the girl to demand that her lover appear to her in his true form. Having promised the girl any gift she desired, Zeus had no choice but to accede to her demand. When he appeared in all his thunderbolt glory Semele literally exploded. Zeus took her unborn child, sewed him into one of his thighs, and gave birth to him later. Dionysos was associated with the fig and the grape, symbols of sex and wine. He was the god of ecstasy and his cult was a mystery religion marked by ritual orgies and bacchanalia. The Dionysian cult was phallocentric. Models of the god's phallus were carried in processions at the Festival of Dionysos at which the great Athenian tragedies were performed, and in other festivals in both Greece and Rome celebrating the god. The Christian church father Augustine of Hippo, in his *City of God* (6:9, 426 CE), wrote that it was Dionysos who was responsible for freeing semen from the male during sex.

Dionysos was particularly related to satyrs and especially to the always erect Silenus, who was said to have been his tutor. Satyrs had donkey's ears and horse's tails. They were commonly depicted in an erect state. They were known for their sexual appetites and were sometimes depicted masturbating, and ejaculating. From satyrs, we take the word 'satyriasis', meaning uncontrollable sexual desire.

The phallocentric aspect of the Dionysian myth was present in the Bacchus myth in Rome as well, Bacchus being the Roman version of Dionysos. Orgiastic bacchanalia rituals in Rome from its earliest days celebrated the phallus. Flying phalli were employed in certain oracular rituals in association with the god Mars (Greek Ares) to ward off evil.

The central Roman myth of the conception of Romulus and Remus is particularly phallic in nature. Plutarch tells how a huge phallus came out of the hearth of the king of Alba Longa and began to fly around the house. An oracle informed the king that the phallus came from Mars to urge him to procreate an heir to his throne. The

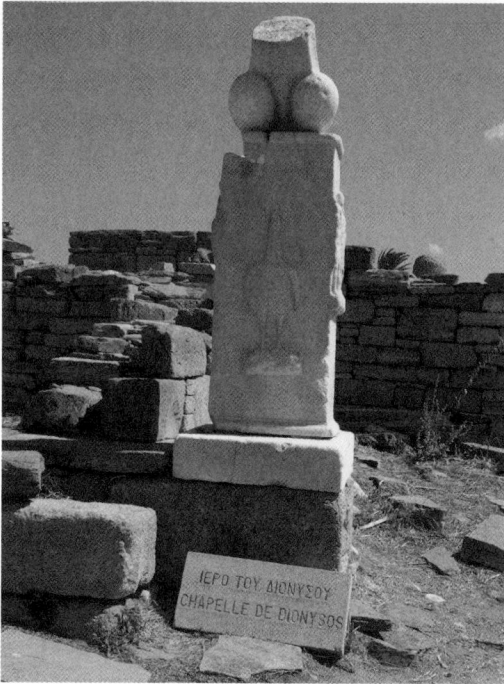

Dionysian phallus at Delos, Greek statue, 300 BCE.

oracle said the king must appease the phallus by presenting it with a virgin for intercourse. The king's daughter refused this role but substituted a slave. The slave woman undertook the task and eventually gave birth to the twin founders of Rome. If sexual relations as depicted in the mythologies of Mesopotamia, Canaan and Egypt are almost exclusively between gods, or gods and humans, in Greek and Roman mythology, as in Hebrew mythology, they frequently involve humans with each other. These relationships reflect many of the same cultural taboos acted out by the gods.

Incest is relatively common in Greek and Roman mythology. Whereas the gods seem not to have been restrained at all by this almost universal taboo, in myths involving humans it inevitably leads to tragedy. The most famous of the incest myths is the one that involves the Theban king, Oedipus. The myth is referred to by Homer and others but its most complete form comes to us in the work of the fifth-century BCE Athenian playwright Sophocles. The Oedipus myth is the source for Freud's 'Oedipus Complex', in which

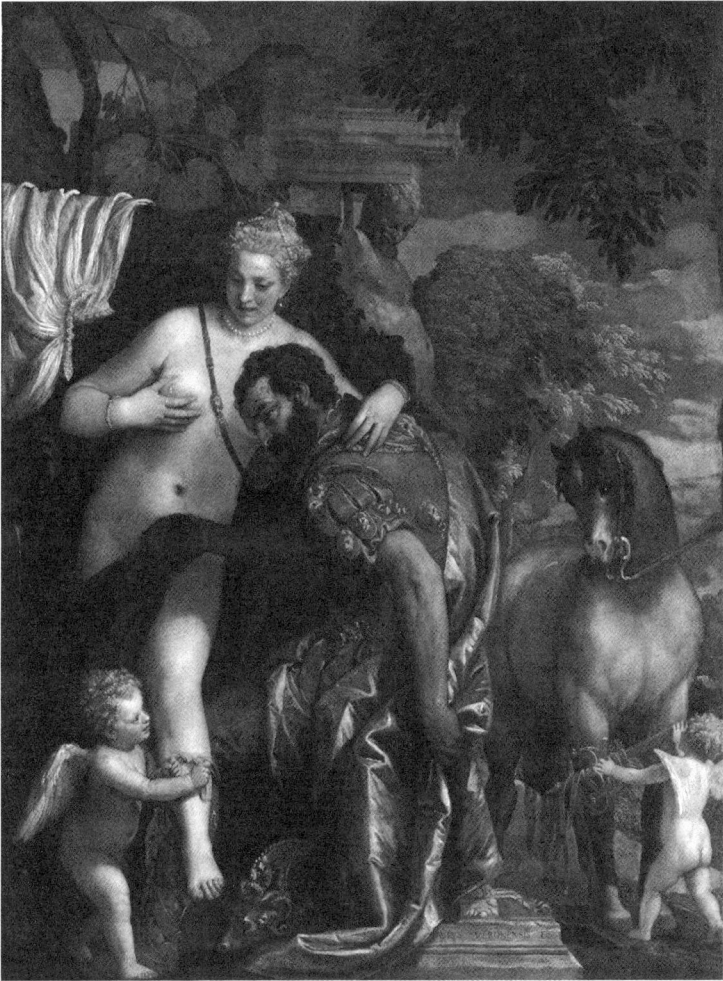

Paolo Veronese, *Mars and Venus United by Love*, 1570s, oil on canvas.

the male child unconsciously desires his mother and wishes for the elimination of his rival father. At the basis of the Oedipus myth told by Sophocles is another sexual myth, the story of Oedipus' father, Laius.

Laius was a descendant of Cadmus, the founder of Thebes and the brother of Europa, the woman whom Zeus, disguised as a bull, abducted. As a young man Laius is forced to go into exile when the throne of Thebes is usurped by others. Laius lives for a while under the protection of King Pelops in the Peloponnesus and while there he rapes the king's son, Chrysippus. Escaping with the boy back to Thebes, Laius became king. Soon he marries Jocasta but is immediately warned by an oracle that he must not have children with her

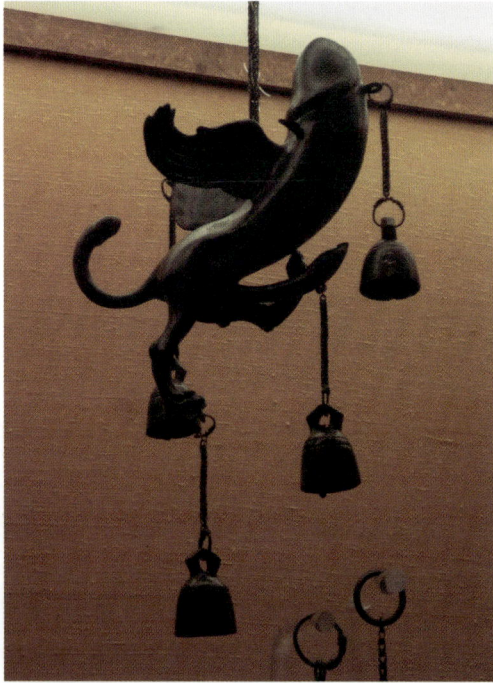

Flying phalli, Roman good luck charms, 2nd century CE.

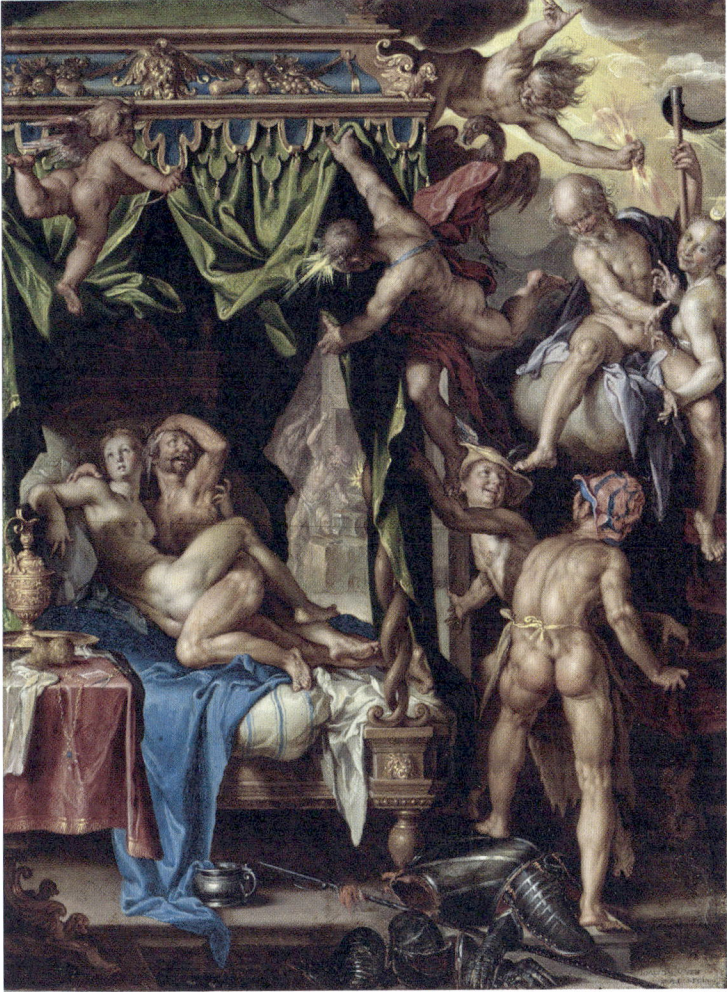

Joachim Anthonisz Wtewael, *Mars and Venus Surprised by Vulcan*,
1604–8, oil on copper.

as his son will one day kill him. Oracles in Greek mythology can never be circumvented, and one night the king becomes drunk and has sex with his wife. The result is Oedipus. Fearing the message of the oracle, the couple leave the child exposed to the elements in the wilderness, but the child is found by a shepherd, who brings him to the royal family of Corinth. The child grows into manhood and is warned by an oracle that he will one day kill his father and marry his mother. Horrified, Oedipus flees Corinth. His adopted parents have never revealed to him that he is not their own child and, naturally enough, he does not want to commit patricide and incest against what he thinks of as loving parents. The gods, however, are apparently determined to have their way with him and he finds himself heading towards Thebes. On the way, he becomes engaged in what is, in effect, a road rage incident with an arrogant man. He fights with the man and kills him. The audience of Sophocles' play knew this background story, including the fact that the man killed was, in fact, Laius, Oedipus' father. Oedipus does not know these facts and proceeds on to Thebes. There he becomes a welcome saviour by answering the riddle of the sphinx that is terrorizing the city. In gratitude, the people make him king (as their former king Laius has never come home from a trip he has taken) and they arrange for him to marry Laius' queen, Jocasta, even though she is much older than Oedipus. Presumably they do this in the interest of political stability. Oedipus and Jocasta have four children – two boys and two girls. Because of the incestuous relationship, of which the married couple is unaware, a plague descends upon the city. Sophocles' play begins with the people begging Oedipus to discover the cause of the plague, and during the events of the play he discovers that *he* is the cause, having killed his father and married his mother.

In another incest myth, the Roman Ovid in his *Metamorphoses* builds on an ancient story about Cinyras, the king of Cyprus, and his daughter, Myrrah. Myrrah's mother has made the mistake of comparing her daughter's beauty to Aphrodite's, causing the goddess to take revenge on the daughter. The vain goddess causes poor Myrrah to fall in love with her father, Cinyras. Myrrah is horrified by her desire, but has sex with her father while he is drunk. This situation is not unlike that of Lot and his daughters. In Freudian psychology, the Myrrah-Cinyras myth would be an example of the 'Elektra Complex', in which the daughter desires her father. The Elektra Complex takes its name from Agamemnon's daughter Elektra, who was so angered by her beloved father's murder that she plotted to have her brother kill their mother. In the case of the Myrrah story, when Cinyras discovers what has happened he pursues his daughter, sword in hand, until she is turned into a Myrrh tree. His and Myrrah's child, Adonis, is born from that tree. Adonis, of course, will become a lover of Aphrodite.

Other incest myths told by Ovid involve Nyctimene, who was raped or seduced by her father and was turned into an owl, and Pelopia who, with her father Thyestes, produced Aigisthos, the lover of Clytemnestra, wife of Agamemnon.

Some sexual taboos in Greek and Roman myth were less significant than incest and were often treated at least somewhat comically. The changing of sex roles was one such taboo. Effeminacy or such practices as cross-dressing among males were not tolerated. The most complex of these myths involved the seer Tiresias.

There are several versions of the Tiresias saga from Hesiod to Ovid, but all begin with his interference with a sex act and all involve his change of gender. It is said that Tiresias came upon two snakes copulating and hit them with his stick. Snakes being sacred to most goddesses beginning in prehistory, the goddess Hera was furious at Tiresias' act and as punishment changed him into a woman ('punishment' because maleness was clearly the preferred gender state in a patriarchal society such as that of the Greeks). As a woman Tiresias had sex with men, had children, and became a priestess of Hera. At the end of his seventh year as a woman Tiresias again came upon copulating snakes but left them alone (or, some say, hit them again). Immediately she was changed back into a man. Unfortunately, Tiresias' transgender experience left him vulnerable to the gods once again. Hera and Zeus were having an argument concerning whether the man or the woman had more pleasure in the sex act. Hera claimed it was the man, Zeus the woman. Tiresias was the obvious person to make a judgement on the issue, and he supported Zeus' position. In a rage, Hera blinded him. As a consolation, Zeus gave the poor man the dubious gift of prophecy.

More comic tales involve cross-dressing on the part of two aggressively male heroes, Herakles and Achilles. In Ovid's treatment of the Herakles (Hercules) myth the great hero exchanged clothes one evening with Omphale, Queen of Lydia, before they went to bed together. Pan (Faunus) lusted after Omphale and snuck into her sleeping place. He lifted her delicate dress only to find the anything but feminine body of Herakles.

As for Achilles, his mother, wishing to avoid her son being drafted into the Trojan War, had him disguised as a girl and placed in the women's quarters at the court of the king of Skyros. Here he was known as Pyrrah, the red-headed girl. He would have avoided the draft had he not been tricked by the wily Odysseus into revealing himself. When Odysseus came to Skyros disguised as a peddler selling women's clothes he was allowed into the women's quarters, where he discovered the hero (who had made one of his girl companions pregnant) by the way he picked up a spear.

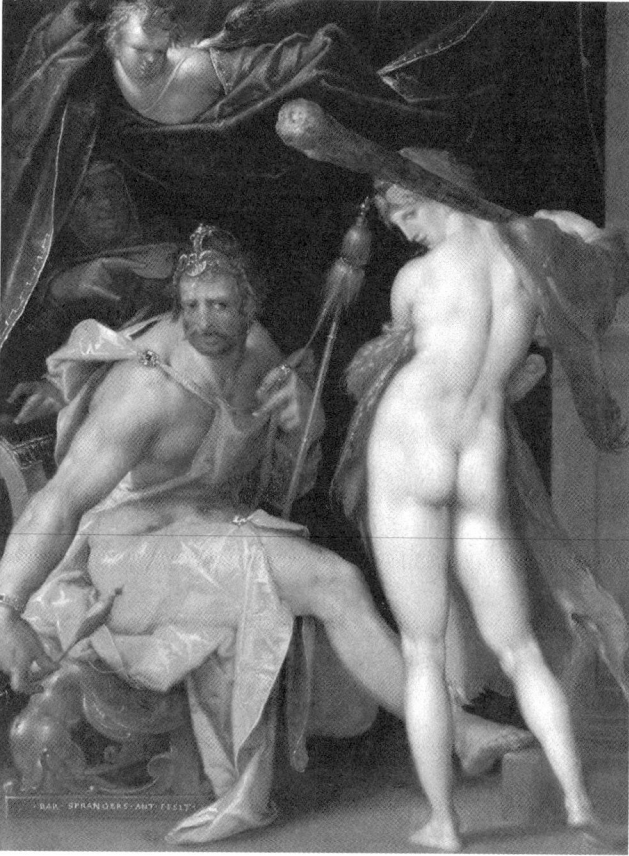

Bartholomeus Spranger, *Hercules and Omphale*,
c. 1585, oil on copper.

In some rare cases, sexual myths involving humans express a
positive, even a romantic, element in sex such as is only rarely found
in the myths of divine sex. Two such relationships stand out, both
related by Homer. The first, in the *Iliad*, is the relationship between
the Trojan hero Hector and his wife Andromache. In a moving scene
before Hector leaves for battle and his probable death, Andromache
tries to dissuade him, arguing in effect for a domestic vision of family

life. Hector, ever the alpha male, obviously has deep and tender feelings for his wife and family but places duty over love. He sends Andromache back to her domestic activities, reminding her that such activities are the place of women while men must attend to civic duty and war. Patriarchy takes precedence over common sense, as it had in the Trojan War itself.

The connection between Odysseus and Penelope in the *Odyssey* is more complex, and sex plays a more important role in that relationship. While Odysseus makes his long and perilous journey back to Ithaca after the Trojan War he finds himself in several sexually charged situations. On the island of Colchys he has an extended affair with the sorceress goddess Circe, and on Ogygia he is detained sexually for several years by the nymph Calypso. It could be argued that these affairs were involuntary, arrangements natural to a hero such as Odysseus. But back in Ithaca, Odysseus' wife Penelope is doing whatever she can, confronted by noble suitors, to remain faithful to a man she might well have assumed to be dead after an absence of many years. Had Penelope given in to a suitor she would have suffered death at the hands of a 'wronged' husband – the fate suffered by the family maids who made the mistake of giving themselves to the pleasure of the suitors. The world of Odysseus, like the world of Hector, was a double-standard male world. After disposing of his enemies Odysseus takes the long-suffering Penelope to the immovable bed he has built, 'her white arms around him pressed as though forever'. Circe and Calypso have no effect on that embrace, and nor did Homer's listeners think they should.

A look back on the sex described in Greek and Roman mythology leads the reader inevitably to two conclusions. Sex among the gods is always outrageous, always self-serving and almost always absurd, and often simply darkly comic. The gods do as they wish.

When gods and humans become involved, the humans always suffer. Humans involved with each other confront in love the limitations established by the gods. It is through the sex myths in Greek and Roman mythology that we experience what can only be called an essentially cynical view of religion, a sense of the painful, even tragic place of humans under the arbitrary and unloving control of these gods.

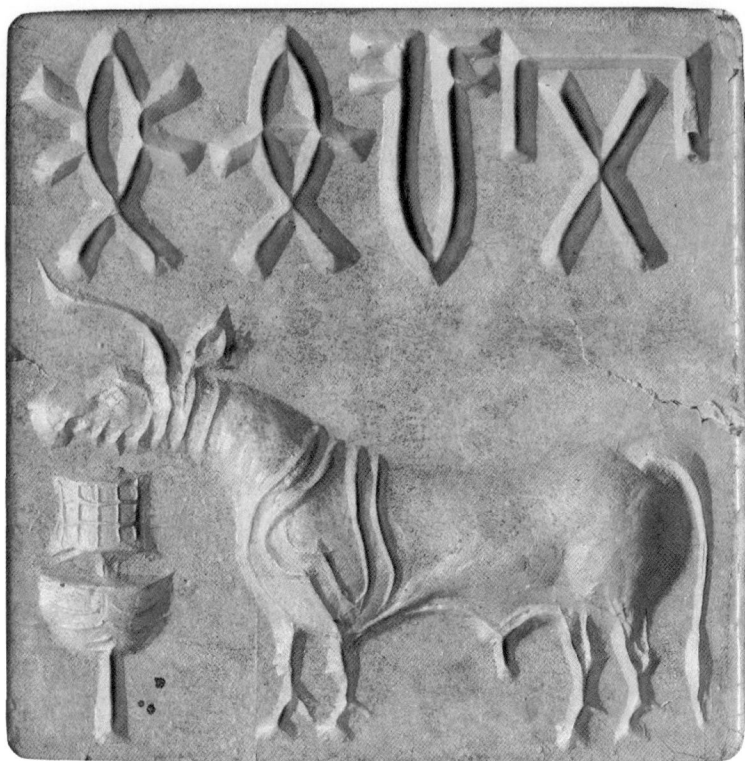

A Brahman bull and possible god symbol, Indus Valley stamp seal, *c.* 2500 BCE.

Five

India

BETWEEN ABOUT 3300 AND 1900 BCE an advanced civilization in what is now India and Pakistan reached its maturity and a level of sophistication that made it comparable to the other three great civilizations with which it was contemporaneous, those of Mesopotamia, Egypt and Crete. Known as the Indus Valley civilization after the Indus River along which it existed or the Harappan civilization after one of its two great cities, Harappa, this civilization emerged from a people who had lived in the valley since perhaps as early as 7000 BCE. The Indus Valley culture, like those of Mesopotamia, Egypt and Crete, with which it almost certainly had trade contacts, had a written language – one that has yet to be deciphered – and a mythology, the basis of which is suggested by language seals and apparently symbolic works of art and ritual.

The Indus Valley civilization had essentially come to an end by 1300 BCE, having either been replaced by invaders or having developed naturally into what we now call the Vedic culture, which would provide the basis for later Indian civilization and Hinduism. In recent years the nationalist movement in India has challenged the traditional scholarly belief that it was Indo-European-speaking people – once called Aryans – from the north who put an end to Indus Valley culture and installed the Vedic culture in its place, although perhaps absorbing some of what they found in the conquered area. There are ample arguments for both the nationalist and Aryan-invasion theories. The Vedic language was a form of Sanskrit, itself an Indo-European language with direct ties, for instance, to Persian, Greek and most European languages. This fact and certain shared mytho-logical themes and character types suggest the invasion. Nationalist scholars argue, however, that figures who clearly became the great gods Vishnu and Shiva already existed in the Valley, suggesting a natural progression from one indigenous culture to another, there being no need of an invasion theory to explain the basis of what became Hinduism.

Whatever the fate of the Indus Valley culture and its place in the development of Hinduism, the archaeological evidence suggests a Harappan mythology in which two sexual aspects were central: the fertile mother goddess and a form of phallus worship. The phallic aspect would remain important in myths of the Vedic period and both the sexual goddess and the phallus would play roles in classical Hinduism.

The Mother goddess as depicted in Indus Valley sculpture is ubiquitous in excavated ruins. Often she reveals herself to us, legs spread, her vulva (yoni) open for sex, and often she is producing offspring. She is the ultimate source of life.

Phallic worship is indicated by the presence of stone columns, somewhat more abstract than the literally depicted male organ (lingam) central to later Shiva worship. Occasionally the phallic symbol and the yoni are joined, perhaps representing wholeness, as in later Hinduism.

Mythology as we have it in textual form begins in India in the Vedic period (c. 1500–500 BCE), the period that precedes the emergence of classical Hinduism. The Vedic texts form the basis of Hindu scripture. These texts are the four Samhitas (mantras, hymns, prayers): the *Rigveda*, the *Yajurveda*, the *Samaveda* and the *Atharvaveda*. The Samhitas, along with associated commentaries and additions known as the *Brahmanas* and *Arayankas* (forest texts) and the somewhat later early philosophical texts, the Upanishads or Vedanta (last Veda), form the totality known as the Vedas. The Vedas are particularly sacred to Hindus as *shruti* ('heard') texts – words from the divine unknown. Other much later sources of Hindu mythology are the *Puranas*, containing legends and folklore, and the great epics the *Mahabharata* and the *Ramayana*. These products of the classical Hindu period are slightly less sacred than the Vedas. They are *smriti* ('remembered') texts and some are associated with specific authors. In both *shruti* and *smriti* literature, sex plays important roles.

The very brief presence of Dyaus (Latin: Father Sky; Greek: Deus, Zeus) and Prithvi (Mother Earth) in the early Vedas (such as the *Rigveda* 1:89.4) suggests a relationship with other Indo-European Sky-Earth personifications – Ouranos and Gaia for instance – who begin the creation process and eventually are replaced in importance by their progeny. The myth of the separation of the original Sky–Earth pair in order that their suffocating union might give way to further creation between them occurs in the mythologies of many non-Indo-Europeans as well – mythologies as widely separate as those of the Sumerians, the Polynesians and many Native North Americans.

It is worth noting also that, as in the Greek creation, Eros (Uncontrollable Desire) emerged from chaos with Gaia in the beginning, so in the *Rig Veda* (10:129.4) Kama (Desire) emerged as Kamadeva (God of Love) at the very beginning of creation. Like the Graeco-Roman Eros/Cupid, Kamadeva is sometimes depicted as a winged male with a bow and arrows. His name was later attached to both the great gods Shiva and Vishnu and Vishnu's avatar Krishna, all of whom play central roles in highly sexualized myths. Kama gives his name to the famous book of Indian erotic love, the *Kama Sutra*, composed in the third century CE. It should be noted, however, that 'Kama' does not refer only to sexual desire; it is a term that can refer to any sensual desire or aesthetic pleasure.

However the sexuality of Hindu mythology is interpreted – as sacred metaphor or as non-erotic symbolism, for example – the fact remains that there is so much explicit sexuality in Indian myth and art as to make the denial of its presence impossible.

Not surprisingly, sex in the Hindu scriptures begins with creation itself. There are several Indian creation myths. These can best be understood not as conflicting versions but as multiple visions of mysterious events that happened before anyone was there to witness them. The *Brihadaranyaka Upanishad* (Sixth Adhyaya, Fourth Brahmana) dating from about 700 BCE addresses creation events as the basis for proper procreative ceremonies. It tells how Prajapati (one of several Prajapatis or creators in Hindu mythology) created a woman and 'revered her below, as one should revere woman below'. The creator's phallus reached out to the woman's 'below' and impregnated her. So the mythical woman's body becomes a symbol for the proper understanding of sex as a consummation of wholeness. The woman's 'below' is the altar of sacrifice; her pubic hair is the 'sacrificial grass'; her labia are the 'fire in the middle'. He who indulges in sexual intercourse, understanding its ceremonial significance, 'turns the good deeds of women to himself' – that is, achieves an element of wholeness. There are dangers for those who do not understand the sacrifice. If, for instance, any semen at all is spilled, whether when one is asleep or awake (that is, through nocturnal emission, coitus interruptus or masturbation), power is lost, semen being a source of power and a necessary element of the sacrifice which is correct intercourse. If semen is improperly spilled, says the Upanishad, it should be retrieved and rubbed between the breasts or eyebrows, accompanied by a mantra:

> This very semen I reclaim!
> Again to me let vigour come!
> Again, my strength; again my glow!
> Again the altars and the fire
> Be found in their accustomed place!

The importance of semen reflects the dominance of the male in proper Vedic intercourse. When the woman has removed the 'clothes of her impurity' the man should approach her and invite her to have intercourse. If she refuses he should bribe her and, failing that, he should strike her and overpower her saying, 'With power and glory I take away your glory.' If the woman then yields she should say to the man 'With power, with glory I give you glory!' Together, then, the man and woman in such intercourse 'become glorious'.

From early on in Vedic mythology there is a theme of conflict as well as union in the act of sex. The woman is even sometimes seen as a demoness. In the *Jaimimniya Brahmana* of *c.* 900 BCE there is the story of the 'long-tongued' demoness who has vaginas in all parts of her body with which to trap the man. This figure has an analogue in the vagina dentata – the vagina with teeth – myth that is found in various cultures around the world. The god Indra deals with the long-tongued demoness by equipping his grandson with multiple penises with which to connect with the woman. Then he destroys her.

In the *Satapatha Brahmana* from the same period, Prajapati divides himself into male and female beings whose intercourse results in various gods, including the beautiful Dawn, whom Prajapati desires. Dawn takes the form of a doe, so Prajapati becomes a stag and impregnates her, an act which results in the world's cattle. The other gods are horrified by this incestuous rape and Rudra – a mythological ancestor of the great god Shiva – shoots Prajapati with his arrows and throws him into the sky.

In still another version it is the creator's wife – his other half – who is horrified by what she considers to be her incestuous relationship with him. She flees from her husband taking various animal forms. He pursues taking the male form of these animals and together they propagate the animal world.

In a much later work, the *Kalika Purana*, the combined creator gods, Brahma and all the Prajapatis, have incestuous designs on the creators' daughter, Dawn. The Lord Shiva is aware of these designs and laughs at the guilty gods. Embarrassed, the gods sweat profusely, and from that sweat a beautiful woman, Rati, is born and becomes the wife of Kama, Kama having, in this version of the story, been born *ex nihilo* from Brahma's mind.

As is evident in other mythologies of the world, incest in creation is a common and, arguably, a necessary act, the difference in the Hindu tradition being that it is recognized as a taboo. As the Vedic scriptures are directly concerned with proper ritual behaviour, it is reasonable that mythological stories should reflect that concern as well as the understanding that Kama (desire), however dangerous, is behind all creative acts.

In classical Hinduism three major gods form a *Trimurti*. These are Brahma the creator, Shiva the Destroyer and Vishnu the preserver, all aspects of the natural process of life and existence itself.

For some Hindus, these gods are simply aspects of the one ultimate reality, Brahman. In practice, however, the three gods, with the Great Goddess Devi taking the place of the somewhat diminished Brahma, are the central figures in three forms of Hindu devotion or *bhakti*. Those who concentrate their devotion on Vishnu are known as Vaishnavas; worshippers of the Lord Shiva are Shaivites; those attached primarily to Devi in her many forms as Shakti, the person-ifications of feminine-based creative energy, are called Shaktas. Each of the primary gods of the original *Trimurti* has his Shakti, his other half, his energizing material power. Brahma's wife is Sarasvati, the founder of language, by which Brahma's eternal creation is articu-lated in time. Vishnu's Shakti is personified as Lakshmi. She is prosperity and good fortune, the worldly expression of Vishnu's power as Preserver of existence. Shiva's Shakti takes several forms. One is Parvati, the fertile wife of the Destroyer. Others are most famously Kali, whose name is the feminine form of *kala* or Time, signifying the necessary devouring principle that dominates the ani-mate world, and the terrifying Durga, the warrior goddess who destroys Mahisha, the monster demon that threatens the universe. Sex plays a major role in relation to each of the members of the original *Trimurti* as well as to Devi/Shakti in her many forms.

Incest and semen dominate one story of the marriage of Brahma and Sarasvati. The *Sarasvati Purana* tells how the god created Sara-svati directly from his semen – that is, from the source of his vitality as a creator. It is said that Brahma became fixated on the personifi-cation of cosmic beauty, Urvasi, and that while he lusted for her he masturbated, collecting his semen in a container. From this semen, the sage Agastya emerged, and Sarasvati emerged from Agastya. Thus, as Athena was born, motherless, of Zeus' head in Greece, in India Sarasvati was the motherless product of her father's semen.

Brahma, like his Vedic mythological ancestor Prajapati/Purusha, admired his daughter's beauty and desired her. Horrified, as Dawn had been earlier, Sarasvati fled from her father until she could no longer resist, and eventually she became his wife.

In the Vishnu-Lakshmi connection the emphasis is not on incest but rather on the concept of the closeness between two beings who depend upon each other in the Shakti relationship. The *Vishnu Purana* emphasizes Lakshmi's loyalty to Vishnu. She is particularly venerated as Sri Lakshmi or simply as Sri, the being who articulates the cosmic reality which is Vishnu. Without Lakshmi's role as action and material energy, Vishnu's cosmic dominance becomes in a sense meaningless. The couple is frequently depicted in erotic union.

The *Vishnu Purana* says that Vishnu and Lakshmi are in a constant state of lovemaking and that this lovemaking is transferred to Vishnu's several avatars (manifestations) who are often matched with Lakshmi avatars. The most famous of these avatar couples is Krishna and Radha. For Vaishnavas, this couple is particularly important – so important that Krishna, as Lord Krishna, takes on a position that seems to be equal to that of Vishnu himself. In the *Bhagavadgita*, for instance, the great philosophical work attached to the epic the *Mahabharata*, he reveals himself as the incarnation of godhead itself, the container of every aspect of existence, as Time and the Universe.

In his human stories, Krishna is more a traditional hero than a god. He is conceived and born miraculouly in Devaki through the agency of Vishnu and the goddess as Maya (holy illusion). Like Jesus and the Persian Zoroaster and other mythical heroes, he is threatened at birth by a wicked king. And like other heroes he reveals his extraordinary nature by performing miraculous deeds as a young child and by killing monsters and helping the 'good side' in the great events of the *Mahabharata* later on. That Krishna is a special

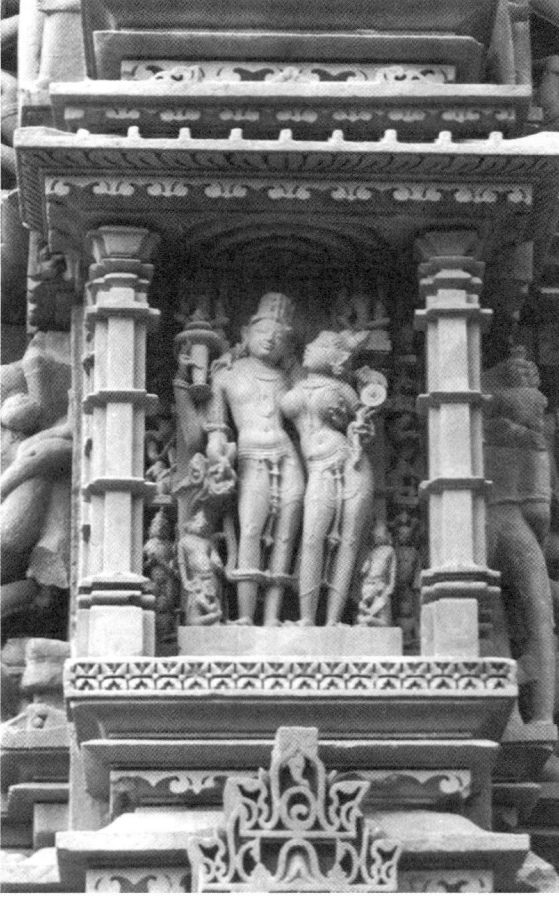

Vishnu and Lakshmi at Lakshmana temple, Khajuraho, *c.* 954 CE.

being his astonished mother understands, when she peers into his open mouth and sees the whole universe there. Although human, Krishna is god incarnate. As a human he is a lover and something of a trickster. But his lovemaking has metaphorical meaning. In one story he takes pleasure from stealing the clothes of his much-loved gopis (cowherds) while they swim. Sitting in a tree above them with their clothes, he will convince the gopis to leave the water with their

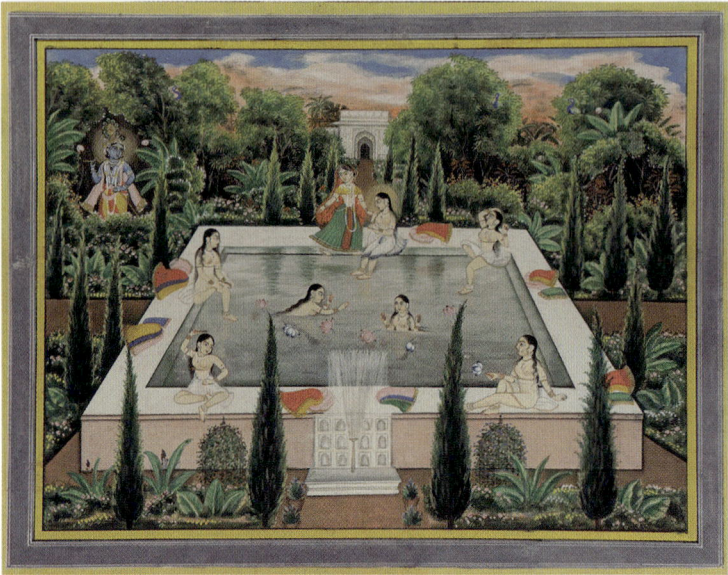

Krishna Watches the Gopis in a Garden Pool, Deccan School miniature, *c.* 1650.

hands together over their heads, signifying in their nakedness their
humility and openness to the god, and in the position of their hands
a state of supplication.

Krishna's true love is the gopi Radha. Krishna and Radha in union
represent the feminine and masculine aspects of godhead. Their
beautifully erotic love bouts reflect those of Vishnu and Lakshmi
and can be seen as an allegory for the human soul's longing for union
with ultimate divinity.

For Shaivites sex is a more explicit and more complex reality
than it is for worshippers of Vishnu. Shiva is inevitably associated
with the concept of the lingam. As noted earlier, the lingam – the
penis as a religious symbol – apparently existed even in the pre-
Vedic Harappan culture. In classical Hinduism it stands as a symbol
of Shiva's power. The *Kurma Purana*, the *Vayu Purana*, the *Shiva
Purana* and the *Linga Purana* tell how Brahma and Vishnu were

arguing over their respective power when Shiva stepped between them in the form of a flaming lingam of which he challenged the other two gods to find the beginning and the end. When the lingam was discovered to be endless, Shiva revealed himself in it and proclaimed dominance, explaining that both Brahma and Vishnu were aspects of *his* supreme divinity. The many versions of this myth are all centred on the Shiva lingam, emphasizing the endless dominance of the Lord Shiva.

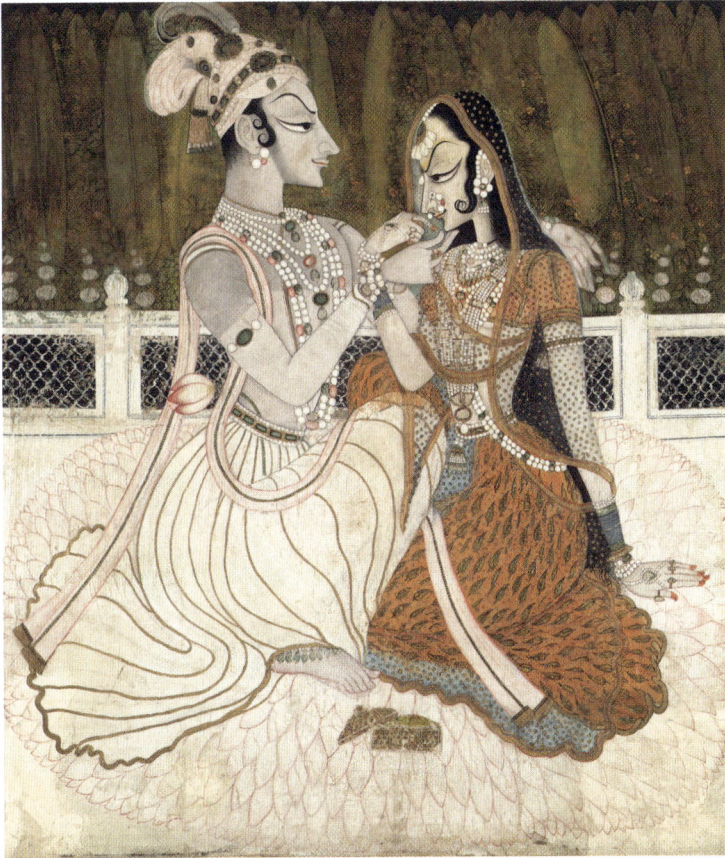

Unknown artist, *Krishna and Radha*, *c.* 1750, painting.

For those who would deny the sexual aspect of the lingam, the lingam is seen simply as a cosmic pillar symbolizing Shiva's power and dominance. Given the explicit phallic nature of so many depictions of the lingam, this interpretation is difficult to accept. This is especially the case when the lingam is associated in both mythology and physical depiction with the concept of the yoni, the yoni being the vulva, which, in conjunction with the Shiva lingam, represents the god's Shakti or creative energy. The *Mahabharata* (13:14) reminds us that all creatures bear the defining marks of Shiva (Mahadeva) – the lingam – and his wife, Uma (Parvati), the yoni. All males have their source in Shiva and all females in Parvati.

The lovemaking activities of Shiva and various forms of Devi make up a great deal of Shiva mythology and of the mythology sacred to the Devi worshippers, the Shaktas, as well as to followers of Tantra. In one story, told in the *Padma Purana*, the sage Bhrigu came to see the god but was denied entry because he was busy making love to Parvati. Angry at being made to wait, the sage cursed Shiva and his Shakti to be worshipped as the lingam and yoni, a form that is ubiquitous in India.

Sages like Bhrigu play a similar role in the *Shiva Purana* when they come upon Shiva beginning to copulate in their forest. Shocked by what they see as an affront, they curse his penis, causing it to fall off. But immediately the phallus travels through the world burning everything before it until the sages agree to find a place for it. That place, Shiva announces to them, was Parvati.

Shiva is not always faithful to Parvati. The *Bhagavata Purana* and the *Brahmanda Purana*, in effect, dispute the dominance of Shiva in the myth of Mohini. In that myth Shiva has sex with Vishnu. Vishnu takes the female form of the beautiful Mohini to beguile the demons and to prevent them from obtaining the nectar of immortality. Hearing of Vishnu's transformation into a woman Shiva convinces him to appear in his female form. At the sight of Mohini-Vishnu Shiva becomes so excited that, despite Parvati's jealousy, he immediately makes violent love with her. Some of his semen escapes and falls onto the ground, becoming silver and gold. When Vishnu returns to his male form he explains that his powers to create illusions cannot be surpassed even by Shiva.

Many of Shiva's sexual encounters occur in myths that are more specifically expressive of the Shakta tradition in which Devi in her various forms is also his mate. For Shaktas, however, the feminine component is the supreme power. Several forms of the Shakta goddess stand out. These are the three wives of the Hindu *Trimurti* and two other forms of Devi, Durga and Kali.

A. K. Ramunajan relates a popular Shakta song that describes Devi as having emerged in creation before the other deities. Very soon she is overcome by her sex drive and creates the god Brahma as a potential lover. Unwilling to sleep with his mother, however, Brahma refuses Devi's advances. Furious, the goddess destroys Brahma with fire generated from her hand. The same fate awaits Vishnu, Devi's second creation. But when he is created, Shiva learns of the fate of Brahma and Vishnu and agrees reluctantly to satisfy Devi's needs. However, when he teaches his new mate his dance of destruction – the dance of life which includes death, Devi incinerates herself with the fire of her own palm. Shiva revives his brothers and together the three gods revive their mother, Devi, who becomes their consorts, Parvati, Lakshmi and Sarasvati.

The Durga story also involves the three wives of the *Trimurti*. Much of it is found in the *Shiva Purana* and in the *Devi Machatmya* or *Durga Saptahati*, which is part of the *Markandeya Purana*. It begins with an act of bestiality. A demon king, Rambha, had sex with a buffalo, and the buffalo gave birth to the buffalo-human Mahishasura, who became a violent potential destroyer of the earth until the three gods of the *Trimurti* agreed to transfer their energy to their consorts, Parvati, Lakshmi and Sarasvati. They then merge these goddesses into one powerful goddess, Durga, who succeeds in defeating the demon Mahishaura, thus saving the world from destruction.

Behind these stories is the idea that the gods themselves require their Shaktis to give material reality and energy to their cosmic essence. Sarasvati gives language, learning and the arts to Brahma's role as creator. She literally makes creation conscious of itself. Lakshmi brings prosperity and beauty and good fortune to Vishnu's role as preserver of creation. As for Parvati, she is the element without which Shiva's power as destroyer is empty, and Shiva and Parvati are often depicted in a sexual relationship.

A particularly complex idea in Shakta and Shaivite theology is that of Ardhanarishvara, a concept of androgyny in which Shiva and Parvati are literally one being, depicted as being divided along a central axis as male and female. In this conception Shiva and his Shakti are an embodiment of eternal wholeness, or Brahman.

Kali is a form of Devi closely related to Durga and for some is synonymous with her. Like Durga, Kali is a consort of Shiva. Sometimes seen as the anger of Parvati and the slayer of monsters, Kali is a Shakti personification of Shiva as the necessary destroyer in a creative process which involves creation, preservation, destruction and renewal. Kali demands the blood sacrifice of male victims. The *Devi Mahatmyam* says she sprang from the head of Durga armed and full of bloodlust. She is often depicted dancing on the prostrate Shiva whose erect phallus reaches up to her as that of Nut had reached up to Geb and Osiris to Isis in Egyptian iconography. For Shaktas the cosmic Shiva is meaningless without the energizing

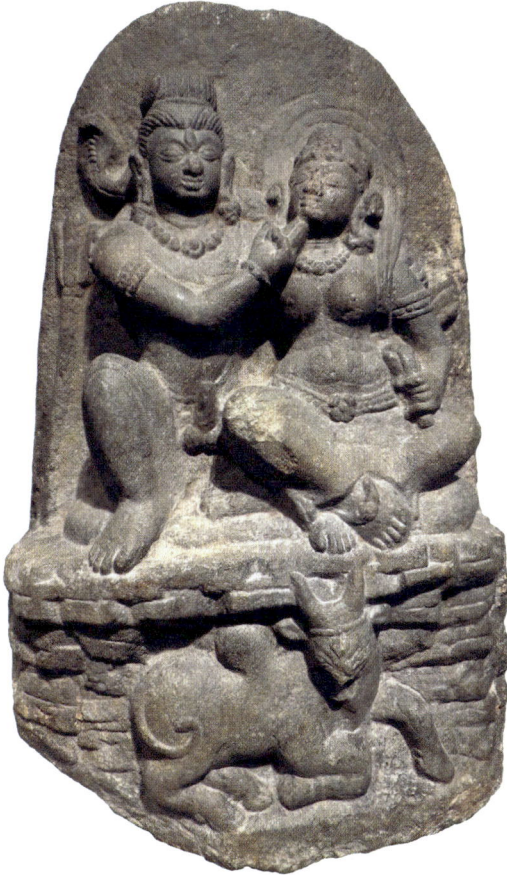

Ithyphallic Shiva with Parvati, 600–700 CE.

force of Kali, whose name, as noted above, is related to the word
for time, the power that devours. Shiva seeks union with his Shakti.
For Shaktas, then, Kali is Kali Ma, the mother of the universe without whom there is no reality.

Kali plays a significant role in the philosophical and ritual
system known as Tantra. When she dances on Shiva his phallus
reaching up to her signifies the longing of men for the goddess, for

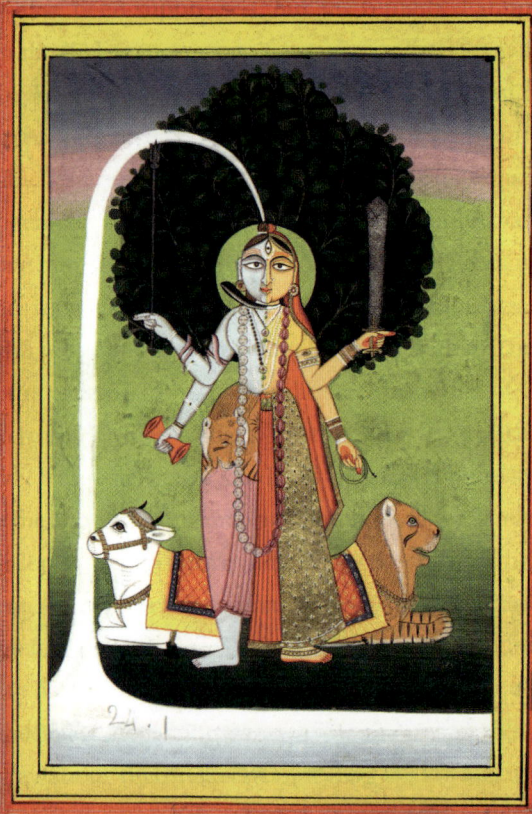

॥सीवपार्वती॥
Seio Parwathy

Ardhanarishvara, the intersex form of Shiva-Parvati,
Shiva-Shakti, 11th century CE.

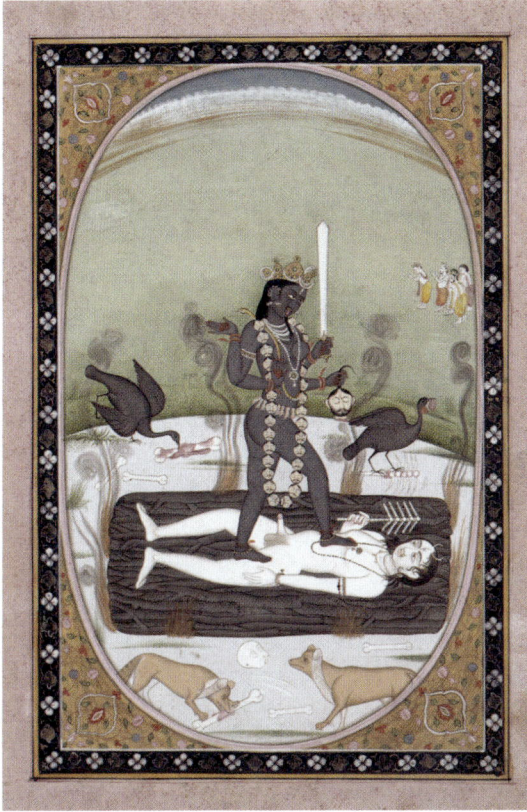

Kali standing on Shiva, *c.* 1800, miniature.

the creative power without which consciousness is inactive. For Shaktas and Shivites of the Tantric persuasion, in which sex is a creative re-enactment of the Shiva-Kali union, Shiva is the divine consciousness of existence while Kali is the creative energy of life. The union of male and female in sex signifies the necessary union of Shiva and Kali.

Much of the Tantric perspective is expressed in the many temple carvings that have confused non-Indians, leading to assumptions that Indian religion is pornographic. An example is the Khajuraho temple complex in Madhya Pradesh, supposedly built in honour of Shiva, who is said to have come there. The temple carvings emphasize the union of male and female, representing not only spiritual union but celebrating Kama, divine-based desire.

Another temple famous for its erotic carvings is the Sun Temple complex of Konark. Created in the thirteenth century and dedicated to the ancient Vedic sun god Surya, its carvings (*maithunas*) signify the union of Shiva and his Shakti, or that of the individual and the divine. The Virupaksha Shiva temple in Hampi celebrates Kama in many different depictions, including dramatic ones of the goddess offering herself to the devotee as the path to the divine.

Kama is most famously referred to in the *Kama Sutra,* the book on erotic love composed in the third century by a man known to us only as Vatsyayana Mallanaga. The Sutra is not primarily a manual of sex positions, though it does deal with that subject. It can be understood, rather, in a spiritual context, as an exploration of one of the four goals of Hinduism: Kama (desire for pleasure and emotional satisfaction), Artha (wealth, success and destiny), Dharma (duty)

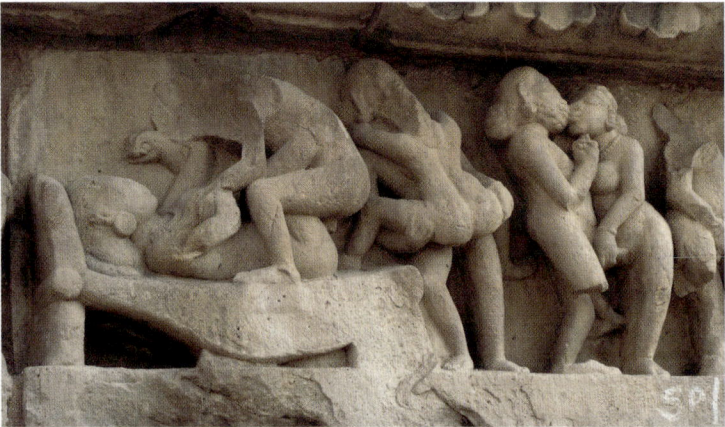

Erotic stone sculpture in a Khajuraho temple, *c.* 954 CE.

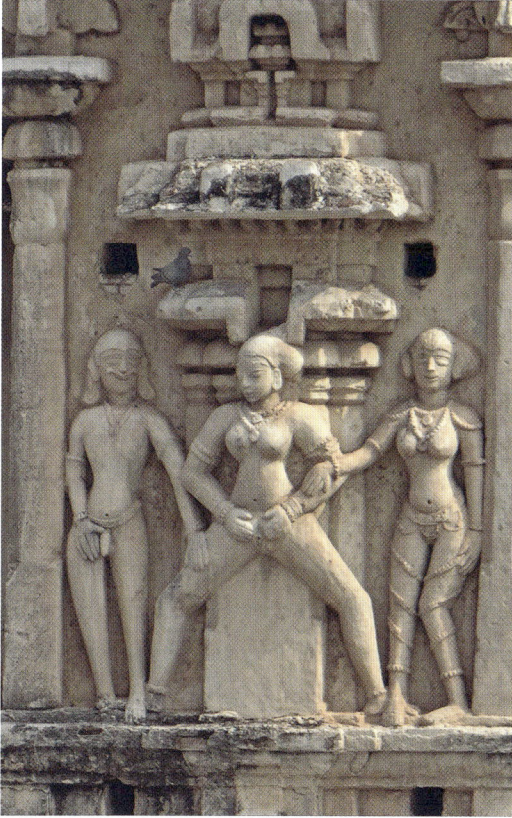

The goddess as Kama at Virupaksha Shiva Temple, 7th century CE.

and Moksha (wholeness, liberation from Samsara, the cycle of life, death and reincarnation). As Wendy Doniger in her *Redeeming the Kamasutra* makes clear, the work speaks to many aspects of Hindu life – such as women's rights and women's sexual pleasure (women should be treated in such a way as to allow them to achieve climax before the man).

What stands out about sex in Indian mythology is the sense of its sacramental aspect, even when taboos are broken and simple pleasure is the goal. Whether the emphasis is on semen, Shiva's phallus, or the Devi's yoni, sex in Vedic and classical Hindu mythology is a sacrificial act and a path to creation or enlightenment. It is very different, for instance, from sex in Greek mythology, in which the purpose seems to be to entertain and to reflect the realities of a highly patriarchal culture. Sex in Hindu mythology is a celebration of one of the central goals of life that exists comfortably and in deep communion with others. Without the fire of Kama there can be no Artha, no Dharma, no Moksha.

Six

Northern Europe: Celts and Norsemen

ELTIC MYTHOLOGY AND Germanic – particularly Norse – mythologies dominated Northern Europe until the arrival there of
Christianity. The Celts are the smallest group of Indo-European
speakers. Scholars disagree as to their origins. Some trace them to
the Beaker and Battle Axe cultures of the third millennium BCE or
to the Urnfield and Tumulus cultures of the second millennium BCE.
A more generally accepted origin is the Central European Hallstatt
culture of the ninth century BCE. Most agree that the fifth century
BCE La Tène culture in Europe, an aristocratic-warrior culture contemporaneous with the high period of Greek civilization, was Celtic.
The Greek historian Herodotus reported that by 500 BCE Celts lived
in most parts of Central and Western Europe. In 390 BCE, Celtic
tribes (*Celtae* or *Galli*) sacked Rome, and in 279 BCE a Celtic tribe
(*Keltoi*) attacked Delphi, and soon after that Celtic tribes (*Galatae*)
had founded Galatia in the area around Gordion, the home of the
mythical King Midas, where Alexander the Great was said to have
destroyed the Gordian Knot. Julius Caesar's Gauls, who divided their
land into three parts, were Celts.

Little is known about the mythology of these Celtic peoples
because the druids in control of Celtic religion disdained written
text for sacred stories. It was not until the first century BCE that Romans

such as Diodorus Siculus, Strabo, Tacitus and most famously Julius Caesar wrote down continental Celtic myths. When they did so they attempted to equate Celtic gods with their own deities, thus corrupting the stories. The solar god Belenus, for instance, was understood to be a version of Apollo. Teutates, a god of war and fertility, was usually thought to be Mars. Taranis, a weather-thunder god, was either Jupiter (Dis Pater or Sky Father) or Pluto, the ruler of the underworld.

Irish Mythology

What we think of today as Celtic mythology is associated primarily with the Celtic tribes of Ireland and Great Britain – Gaels in Ireland and Scotland, the Cymri, Brythons and the Belgae, whose descendants settled in Wales and Cornwall (as well as in Brittany). Celts reached Ireland and Britain perhaps as early as the sixth century BCE. In some areas these Celts were attacked by the Romans and much later by Germanic peoples (Vikings or Norse, Angles and Saxons). Insular- as opposed to continental-Celtic mythology was not written down until the sixth century CE when Irish monks attempted in their manuscripts to preserve the traditions of their homeland by recording ancient myths. But again, as on the Continent, these retellings were corrupted. In this case, many centuries had passed since the Celtic arrival, and the monks naturally attempted to some extent to reconcile the pagan mythology with the beliefs of their own religion. One result of that attempted reconciliation is the absence of much explicit sexuality.

Insular Celtic mythology as it has come down to us, because of the natural corruption of the tales by time and ideology, is best thought of not as Celtic mythology but as separate but related mythologies associated with the Celtic peoples who settled in specific Celtic lands. Thus, realistically we have, for instance, Irish mythology and Welsh mythology, which have little in common with the mythology of the Romanized continental Celts and differ significantly from each other.

Of all the Celtic mythologies, Irish mythology is most fully known. It has been argued that by the middle of the seventh century most of this mythology had been written down by the monks in what is called the *Tech Screpta* writings preserved on carved sticks. But this body of work was looted by Vikings beginning in the eighth century. It was not until the twelfth century that monks at Clonmacnois, Glendalough, Terryglass and elsewhere compiled the great mythological texts: the *Lebhor na hUidre* (Book of the Dun Cow) and the *Lebhor na Nuochongbhala* or *Lebhor Laignech* (Book of Leinster). Later came the *Great Book of Lecan*, the *Yellow Book of Lecan*, the *Book of Ballymote* and the *Book of Fermoy*, all based on much earlier texts. Other important texts are the *Cath Maige Tuired* (The Battle of Mag Tuired) and a later account known as the *Second Battle of Mag Tuired*. In addition to these works are heroic tales collected in the Ulster or Red Branch Cycle. The sources for this cycle are the twelfth-century manuscripts and the *Yellow Book of Lecan*. The primary narratives of the Red Branch Cycle are the great Irish epic, the *Táin Bó Cúailnge* (The Cattle Raid of Cúailnge), and the lesser-known *Táin Bó Fraoch* (The Cattle Raid of the Fraoch). Other heroic tales, collectively known as the Fenian or Ossianic cycle, have their source in the twelfth-century *Acallam na Senórach* (Colloquy of the Ancients). The mythology dealing with the origins of Irish culture is contained in a compilation called the *Lebhor Gabhala Éireann* (Book of Invasions), the most complete version of which is that of Míchael Ó Cléirigh in the seventeenth century.

The mythical invasions began, according to most of the Christian redactors, with the arrival of Noah's granddaughter Cesair or, some say, of Banbha, one of the eponymous queens who stood as symbols in themselves of Irish sovereignty. According to the Cesair version, the great biblical flood destroyed all the invaders except for Cesair's husband Fintan, who saved himself by turning himself into a salmon. Despite this trickster-like shape-shifting act, Fintan does not share the usual highly active sexuality of tricksters elsewhere.

The followers of Partholon came next and began clearing land. But after fighting the invading violent Fomorians (Fomhoire), who came from the sea, they all died of a plague. Nemed (Nemhedh) then arrived with four women, who produced the Nemedians. These people continued the land clearing, and they fought the Fomorians but were defeated by them and treated so badly that they left the island. Some sources say the Nemedians returned in a later invasion as the Firbolg (Fir Bholg) or 'Bag Men', a name stemming from their having been forced to carry bags of soil during their exile in Thrace. The Firbolg – perhaps a version of actual pre-Celtic people in Ireland – divided the island into five provinces or fifths (coiceds). These provinces, basic to Irish mythology and history, are Ulster, Connaught, Munster and Leinster, all coalesced around Mide (Meath) where, according to the mythic history, the sacred kingship was eventually established with its seat at Tara. The sovereignty of the sacred monarch was based on his association with the land's fertility, represented by three eponymous queens, Ériu, Banbha and Fótla, personifications of sovereignty itself. Phallic stones such as the Lia Fáil or Stone of Destiny placed on a sacred mound at Tara perhaps signify among other things the king's role in fertilizing the land.

It was the Tuatha Dé Danann (People of Danu), the next invaders, who are said to have brought the phallic stones and the female statuettes known as the Sheela na gig to Ireland. These were deities who were descended from a version of the great Indo-European mother goddess Danu. Two hills in Kerry to this day are called the 'Paps of Anu [Danu]'.

Goddesses in general play an important role among the Tuatha. These are in the general tradition of fertility or mother goddesses, the Matres, who offer their bodies freely to all, including mortals, and who can take form as the tripartite goddess or other specific figures – such as the Sheela na gig, or even the more ambiguous Morrigan,

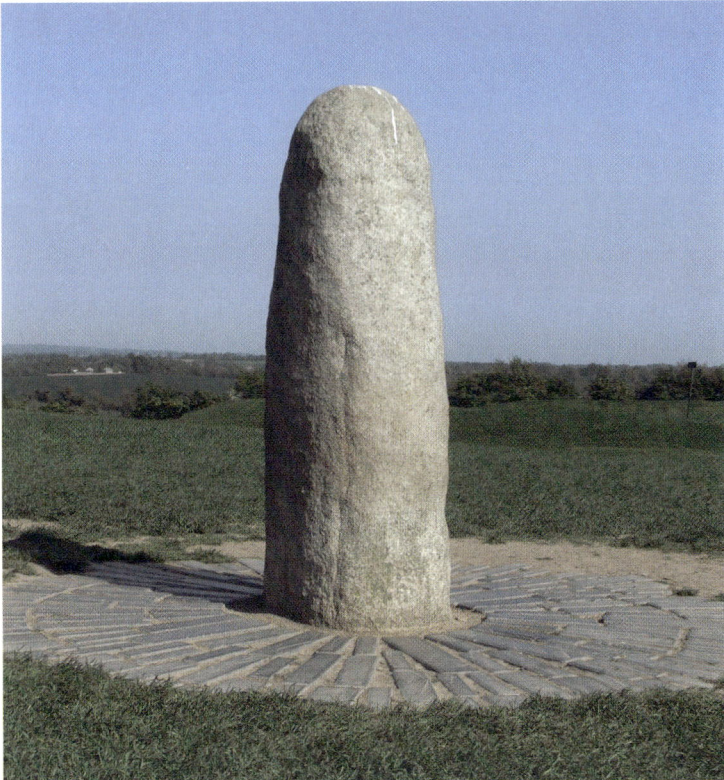

Lia Fáil, the coronation stone at Tara, also known as the Stone of Destiny, possibly 12th century.

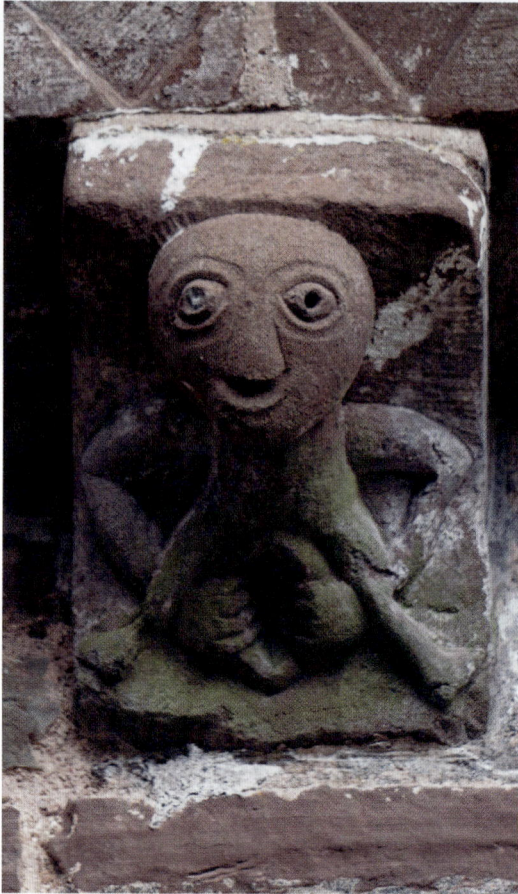

Sheela na gig statuette, probably 12th century CE.

who in the *Second Battle of Mag Tuired* has sex with the leader of the Tuatha, the Dagda or All Father, who comes upon her bathing. Their lovemaking place is known as 'The Bed of the Couple'. It was said that during their lovemaking Morrigan warned the Dagda of an imminent landing by the Fomorians.

Another more explicit but comically scatological sexual event involving the Dagda occurs later in the *Second Battle*. The Dagda had gone on a diplomatic mission to ask the Fomorians for a truce. The Fomorians agreed but tricked him into eating a huge amount of porridge, which caused his belly and 'rump' to become so bloated that he could hardly walk. As he headed for home he left 'the track of Dagda's club', a euphemism for his extremely long penis. On the way, he came across a good-looking young woman and desired her, but the swelling of his belly made him impotent. The mysterious woman made fun of him, hurled him into a hole in the ground and beat him so badly that his bowels opened violently. Finally, the Dagda rose and the woman demanded that he carry her on his back. The Dagda did what he was told but put three stones in his belt. The stones fell from his belt and, according to the text, are commonly thought to have been his testicles. The girl on his back struck him on the rump and in so doing revealed her 'curly pubic hair'. The Dagda then became potent and the pair stopped to make love. Their lovemaking is marked at Beltraw Strand.

One of the Dagda's children was Brigid, who is perhaps the mythological ancestor of the British Brittania and who in Christian times became St Brigid of Kildare, associated with poetry, fertility and vestal virgins, or nuns. In Scotland, she is celebrated as the midwife of the Virgin Mary and the foster-mother of Jesus.

The goddess takes many different forms. She is Macha or Nemain and sometimes Morrigan, and was married to another Tuatha king, Nuada, who lost his arm during the first battle of Mag Tuired against the Firbolg. His arm was replaced with a silver one by the medicine god Dian Cecht. But Nuada and Macha were both killed during the second battle of Mag Tuired, in which the Fomorians were defeated by the Tuatha.

The couplings between Morrigan, or other forms of the Matres, and the Tuatha kings is a pre-figuring of the Celtic understanding of the importance of the union between the Irish king at Tara and the fertility of the land itself represented by the Matres, the queens represented in their various forms.

The final invasion in the story of Ireland's founding is that of the Gaels or Celts, represented by the Milesians, the sons of Mil. The monks who wrote the *Book of Invasions* saw the Milesian invasion in light of the biblical Book of Exodus, telling how the Milesians, led originally by Mil, who died during the voyage to Ireland from Spain, were guided by the mystical prophet-poet Amairgen. The poet, like Krishna in the *Bhagavadgita*, seems to have contained the land within himself, and, in a sense, he sang it into existence through his poetry. The Milesians confronted the Tuatha, and on their way to Tara to meet the three Tuatha kings there, they met the three eponymous goddesses who convinced the invaders to name the country after them. Thus, the land became Éire, after the goddess Éire (Ériu), whose name achieved dominance over the names of the goddess's other embodiments, Banbha and Fótla.

The peace settlement between the Tuatha and the Celts left the Celts in control of the land above ground and the Tuatha in control of the world below ground. The Tuatha in Irish legend now became a fairy people, the 'little people' or *Sidh*, who lived in *sidhe*, mounds found all over Ireland. Now Ireland was ready for the heroic sagas telling of the lives of heroes, such as Queen Medb (Maeve), Cúchulainn and Finn. These figures, being more 'human' than any of the mythical invaders, were also, despite their Christian redactors, more overtly sexual.

Queen Medb of Connaught is the instigator of the events of the great Irish epic the *Táin Bó Cúailnge*, in which she is the hero Cuchulainn's primary rival in the war over her attempt to gain possession of the Brown Bull of Cúailnge.

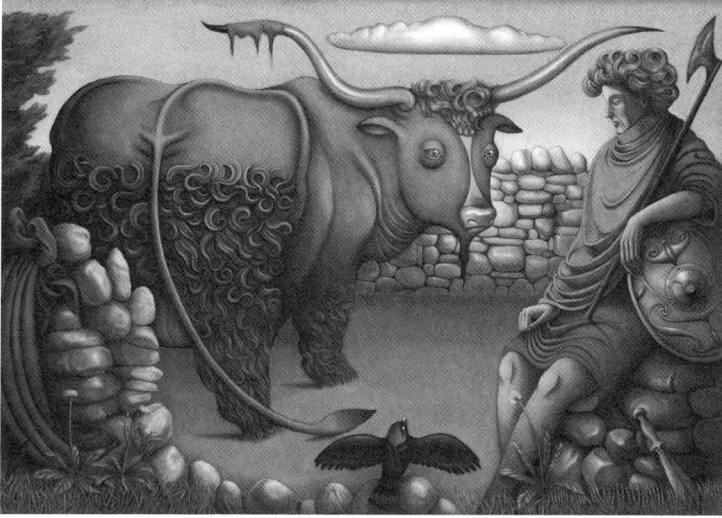

Karl Beutel, *Cúchulainn and the Bull*, 2003, oil on canvas.

The bull is a highly symbolic animal in Irish mythology as, indeed, it is in prehistoric mythologies in the Middle East and in the mythologies of Mesopotamia, Canaan, Greece and India. The bull is always a male fertility figure closely linked to a female – usually a goddess – who represents the fertility of the land. In the *Táin,* Medb's desire for the bull points back to her original role as a great battle goddess who represents Sovereignty. Kings of Ireland in sexual union with Medb symbolized the union of the Celtic sacred kingship with the land. The kingship of the Tuatha god and king Lugh, who succeeded the Dagda, is represented by his sexual union with the goddess, in this case Rosmerta, as 'Sovranty'. In her positive sexual aspect Medb resembles the Sumerian Inanna in her sexual union with the king, Dumuzi. In the sagas, Medb mated with several kings and is herself a version of 'Sovranty'. She is not always a positive figure, however. Her obsession with the sacred bull is reminiscent of the Minoan Pasiphae's more extreme obsession with the great white bull of Poseidon. Medb is ruthless as a battle queen, as is her mythological sister Morrigan, and like her earlier mythological sister, the Babylonian Ishtar and countless other love goddesses of myth, she has elements of the femme fatale.

The greatest of the Irish heroes was Cúchulainn. His mother was Dechtire, a daughter of the druid Cathbad, and the Tuatha love god Aonghus. She was impregnated by the god Lugh, who became a mayfly and flew into the young woman's drink. From this immaculate conception, associating him with so many heroes of myth, Cúchulainn was born. As a seventeen-year-old he joined Ulstermen in their battle with Queen Medb over the Brown Bull of Cúailnge. He was so successful in battle that the enemy queen, Medb, here as the mythical femme fatale, became enamoured of him and hoped to seduce him into becoming her follower. She failed in this attempt, but that did not deter the Great Goddess in her form as Morrigan from making a similar attempt, in this case more overtly sexual. Appearing to the hero in a red dress on a horse, she claimed it was she who had enabled him to be so successful in battle, and she demanded love in return. Like Gilgamesh refusing Ishtar's advances, Cúchulainn perhaps made a fatal mistake here. Morrigan became not the sovereign ground for sacred kingship but a battle goddess and femme fatale who would eventually celebrate the hero's death – a death planned by Medb and executed by her followers – by landing on his dying shoulder as a raven.

A footnote to sexuality in the Cúchulainn saga which resembles a perhaps equally disputable footnote to the David and Jonathan story in the Bible is that of his relationship with Ferdia. During a *Tain* battle Medb tries to trick Cúchulainn by sending out his boyhood friend and foster-brother Ferdia to fight him. When the two approach each other, Cúchulainn reminds Ferdia that they had once

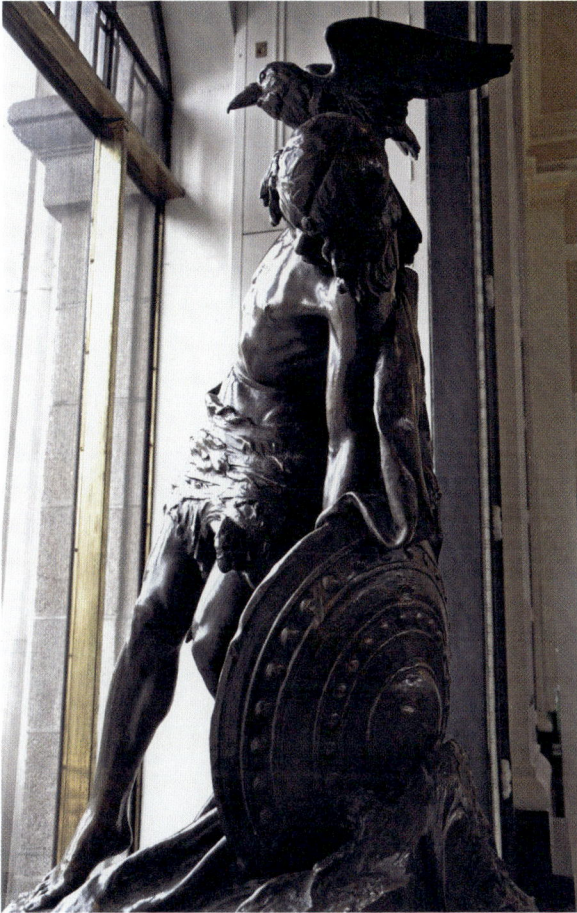

Oliver Shepherd, *The Death of Cuchulainn* (with Morrigan as a raven), 1911, bronze sculpture.

been 'companions of the heart . . . men that shared a bed'. After reluctantly fighting and killing Ferdia, Cúchulainn laments, 'I loved the noble way you blushed, and loved your fine, perfect form. I loved your blue clear eye, your way of speech, your skilfulness.'

Welsh Mythology

Celtic mythology in Wales is even more corrupted by later influences than that of the more isolated Ireland. There are, of course, oral sources, including attributions to the mythical poet-prophet Taliesen, the Welsh equivalent of the Irish Amairgen. But Welsh mythology as we know it is essentially contained in the medieval collection known as the *Mabinogion* or *Mabinogi*, found in two fourteenth-century manuscripts, the *White Book of Rhydderch* and the *Red Book of Hergest*. The *Mabinogion*, divided into four 'Branches', is probably based on oral narratives that took literary form in the eleventh and twelfth centuries under strong Christian influence. The Four Branches are concerned with the Children of Don, the Welsh equivalent of the Tuatha De Danaan. Other than the Branches there are a group of independent tales, several involving King Arthur's court.

As in Irish mythology, sex – certainly explicit sex – plays a relatively minor role in the *Mabinogion*. In keeping with the Celtic tradition, however, the marriage union of kings with fertility goddesses does remain a dominant theme. In the First Branch, King Pwyll is sitting on his throne mound when a beautiful woman rides by on a white horse. Immediately captivated, he gives chase to the woman, who finally stops, revealing herself as the goddess Rhiannon, perhaps the Welsh form of the Gaulish horse goddess Epona. After several near disasters, Pwyll and Rhiannon are married, and a son, the Welsh hero Pryderi, is born.

The Second Branch of the *Mabinogion* also concerns marriage, this one a tragic union between Branwen, the brother of the giant Bran, both children of the Welsh King Llyr (Lir, Lear) by Iwweriadd (Ireland) or by Penardun, the daughter of the Mother Goddess Don. Branwen herself is sometimes considered a love goddess. She is betrothed to King Matholwch of Ireland, a marriage that points back to the tradition of the King of Ireland in union with the goddess as Sovereignty. In fact, Branwen gives birth to Gwern, who is given the title of 'Sovranty' of Ireland, signalling a union of the Celtic lands of Ireland and the Wales of Branwen and Bran. The union deteriorates when the evil Efnisien brings about enmity between the Irish people and Branwen, causing the giant Bran to form a bridge between the two countries to allow an invasion of Ireland. After the ensuing war, only five pregnant Irish women, seven Welshmen and Branwen, who soon dies of a broken heart, are left.

The Third Branch also concerns marriage, between Pryderi and Cigva and Pryderi's mother, the widowed goddess Rhiannon, and a son of King Llyr, the wise Manawydan. These marriages are plagued by malicious forces that would deny the proper union of king and goddess, but eventually the family prevails.

The Fourth Branch concerns sexual relationships, this time among the gods, the Family of Don themselves. It is a story of incest, deception and misogyny more in keeping with the tales of the Greek gods than of the myths usually associated with the Celtic deities. The god of wealth, Math, insists upon having a virgin's lap as a footstool when he is not at war. Gwydion and Gilfaethwy, two of the sons of Don, steal the virgin, and Gwydion tries to use his sister Aranrhod as a substitute. It is soon discovered that Aranrhod is no virgin. As she steps over Math's sword in a test of her virginity, the sea god Dylan drops from her womb and soon after that she gives birth to another child who turns out to be the result of her incestuous relationship with her brother Gwydion. This child is the hero Lleu Llawgyffes, whom Aranrhod swears will never marry into a 'race now on earth'. Gwydion circumvents this curse by creating the beautiful Blodeuwedd from flower blossoms broom, and

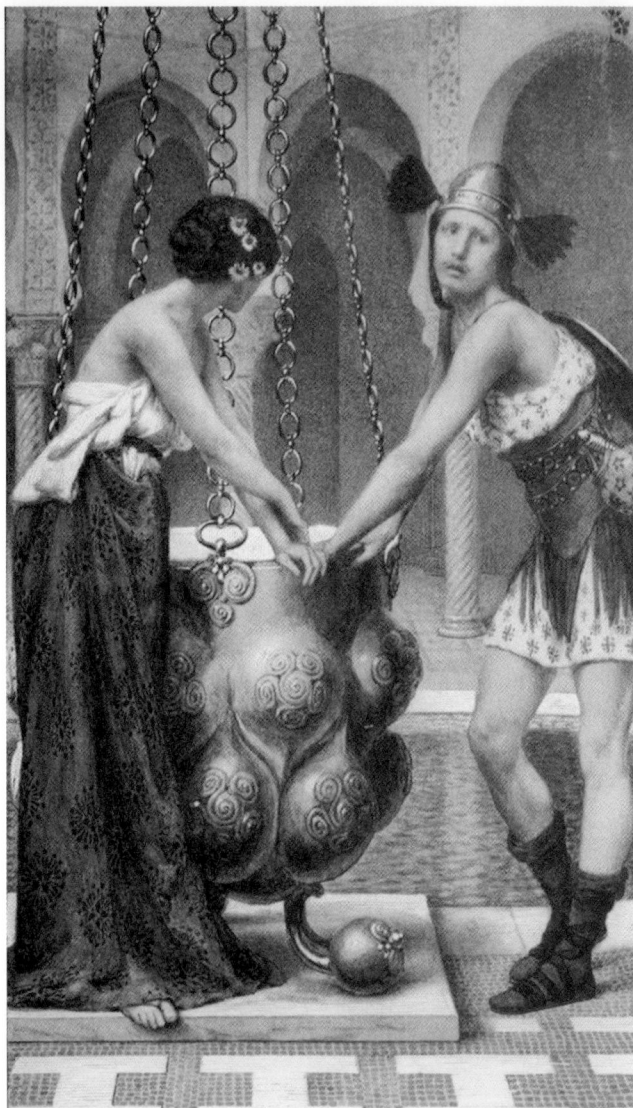

Albert Herter, 'Pryderi and Rhiannon', illustration from
Tales of the Enchanted Islands of the Atlantic (1899).

the meadowsweet. She becomes Lleu's wife, but falls in love with Gronw of Penllyn and the lovers plot to kill Lleu. After they succeed in the murder, Gwydion brings Lleu back to life. Lleu kills Gronw and turns Blodeuwedd into an owl.

The Arthurian tales of Welsh mythology as contained in the last sections of the *Mabinogion* are derived primarily from the twelfth-century romances of Chretien de Troyes, whose sources were likely earlier Breton and Welsh versions. The story of Geraint and Enid, in which a lover mistrusts his beloved, ends in the traditional Celtic fashion in which the beloved proves herself and thus brings her lover back into the fold of her sovereignty.

Other aspects of the Arthurian myth come from the early ninth-century *Historia Brittonum* by Nennius, the *Historia regum Britanniae* by Geoffrey of Monmouth and the fifteenth-century *Le Morte d'Arthur* by Sir Thomas Malory. Gradually, the Arthurian saga became part of the Christian system as applied specifically to Great Britain as a whole rather than specifically to Wales. Thus, there is the tradition of Joseph of Arimathea's bringing to Britain the holy grail (Sangreal), the vessel used at Jesus' Last Supper, which was the goal of the quests of the Knights of the Round Table. Joseph's staff was said to have given forth the holy thorn tree at Glastonbury Abbey. The belief that Jesus himself came to England was made popular in William Blake's words from the poem 'Milton', words that became the hymn 'Jerusalem':

> And did those feet in ancient time
> Walk upon England's mountains green?
> And was the holy Lamb of God
> On England's pleasant pastures seen?

The monks at Glastonbury Abbey, where so much of this Christian lore relating to Arthur developed, always maintained that 'the Once and Future King' was buried there where a stone to this day claims to mark the spot.

Despite the Christian influence on the Arthurian tales, there is a significant amount of sexuality in them, almost all of it viewed negatively. Arthur's conception itself is a perversion of the usual miraculous conception of the universal hero. Malory and others relate how Uther Pendragon of Britain was assisted in his struggle against the invading Saxons by the Duke of Cornwall (Cornwall being a Celtic land). But when Uther fell in love with the Duke's beautiful wife Igraine and did not hide his affection, the Duke hid her away at the Castle of Tintagel on the coast. While the Duke was away at war, Uther, with the help of the magician Merlin, managed to get into the castle and into Igraine's bed, disguised as the Duke. The result was Arthur's conception. The Duke of Cornwall was killed that night. Inevitably here one remembers the story of King David's taking possession of Bathsheba by sending her husband off to war to be killed.

Other perversions play a part in the Arthurian mythology. Incest is a prime example. According to Malory, Morgause, Arthur's half-sister, unaware of her relationship to Arthur, visited his bed, and the result was the conception of Mordred, who would become the king's fatal enemy. It has become popular to conflate Morgause with her sister Morgan le Fay, who was often the king's enemy. According to some versions of the story, Mordred seized the crown while Arthur was off fighting the Romans and then married the king's wife, Guinevere. Others say that the queen refused Mordred and escaped to the Tower of London. Still others, including Chretien de Troyes, tell the more popular tale of the queen's affair with Lancelot. The

Lancelot-Guinevere relationship was discovered, some say by Mordred and other knights who came upon them in bed, leading to the exile of Lancelot and the hiding of the adulterous queen in a nunnery. The ultimate result of the relationship was the undermining of the fellowship of the Round Table.

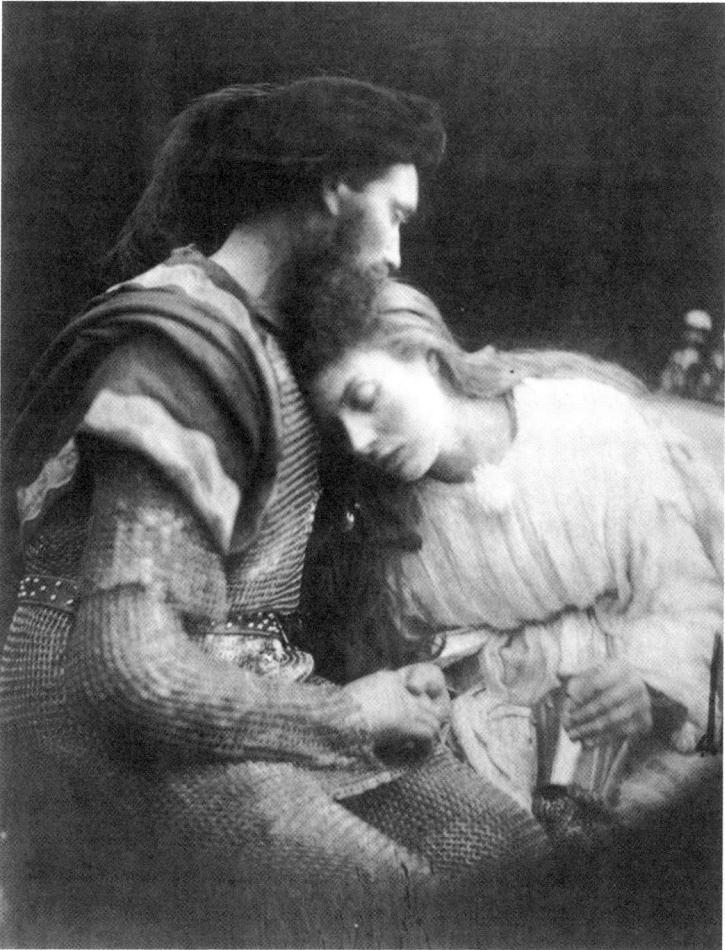

Julia Margaret Cameron, *The Parting of Sir Lancelot and Queen Guinevere*, 1874, albumen silver print.

The Lancelot-Guinevere story was probably influenced by an earlier folktale involving the adulterous relationship between Tristan and Iseult, and an even earlier Irish one involving Naoise and Deirdre. In the Irish story King Conchobar plans to marry Deirdre, the most beautiful woman in Ireland – this despite a prophecy that Deirdre will cause the destruction of Ireland. Deirdre, however, falls in love with the handsome courtier Naoise and they run off together. The king lures them back with a promise of amnesty but kills Naoise and makes Deirdre his wife. Deirdre later commits suicide. All this leads indirectly to the great war described in the *Tain Bo Cuailnge*. In the Tristan and Iseult story, Tristan is bringing Iseult, as promised, to King Mark of Cornwall as a wife. But given a magic love potion by Iseult he falls in love with her and continues an adulterous relationship with her until inevitable tragedy overcomes the lovers.

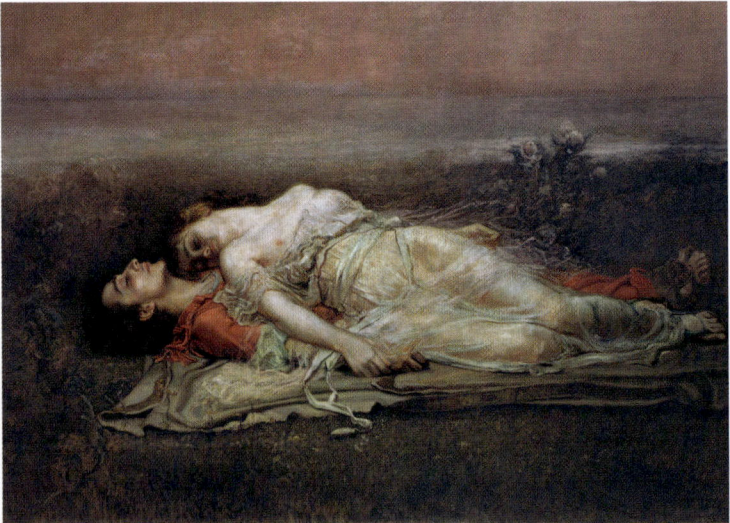

Rogelio de Egusquiza, *The Death of Tristan and Iseult*, 1910, oil on canvas.

In these tales, physical love, often complicated by taboos, is pitted against loyalty to the king, to whom the young woman in question 'belongs'. In a sense, then, the tales question the whole Celtic concept of the king in union with the woman as 'Sovereignty' and interject a whole new vision of sexuality. The Celtic sovereignty ideal relating to women recalls the Hindu concept of the god and his Shakti – represented by a goddess in union with whom his essence gains energized material power. Once the woman in the equation becomes a femme fatale, as in the case of Medb, Morrigan, Morgause or Morgan le Fay, the ideal is shattered. It could be argued that chivalry was a means of preserving the proper union. A man could 'worship' a woman and depend on his connection with her to guide him in his life. But sex with the woman would break the chivalric code that assumed sexual desire, but desire dominated by Christian spiritual longing and the idealization of chastity. The sex act itself in this context would cause dissolution in society, as in the cases of Lancelot and Guinevere and Tristan and Iseult. A perhaps more cynical and less romantic perspective of the Celtic view of the woman as Sovereignty derives from the fact that the primary means of preserving property rights was marriage. Land meant power and land often went with the woman to the man seeking power.

Norse Mythology

The Germanic peoples, including the people of Scandinavia and various tribes in Northern Germany, emerged from the Iron Age Jastorf culture at least as early as the sixth century BCE.

Norse mythology – the mythology of the Vikings, the Scandinavians and Icelanders who raided the rest of Europe between 780 and 1070 CE – is the best preserved of the mythologies of the Germanic peoples. The Germanic mythology further south, contained in medieval works such as the Anglo-Saxon *Beowulf* or the German epic the *Nibelungenlied*, were written by Christianized writers, there having been no written Germanic language there other than a limited runic script before the coming of the new religion. Most of these Germanic people had adopted Christianity by the sixth century CE. Christianity, however, was slow in coming to the far north. It was not until the year 1000 that the Icelandic Assembly voted to replace the old religion with Christianity. There are reports of sacrifices to the Norse god Odin at Uppsala in Sweden as late as 1070. Thus, the great redactors of Norse mythology, the Danish historian Saxo Grammaticus (1150–1216) and the Icelandic poet and statesman Snorri Sturluson (1179–1241), were significantly closer to their subject than, for instance, the author of the *Nibelungenlied* in Germany. Furthermore, Saxo and Snorri were genuinely committed to preserving knowledge of the ancient pre-Christian culture in their world. The result was reasonably uncontaminated redactions.

It is on Snorri especially that we most depend for our knowledge of Norse mythology. A gifted researcher and historian, Snorri made use of early material collectively known as the *Poetic Edda* to retell the ancient tales in his *Prose Edda*, which he meant to be used by poets and scholars as a handbook and guide to the old mythology. The sections of the *Poetic Edda* most used by Snorri were the *Voluspa*, the story of the beginning and ending of the world, the *Grimnismal*, in which the high god Odin, the All Father, speaks, and the *Havamal*, which contains the strange tale of the self-hanging of the high god. He also used stories contained in skaldic poems, skalds being Norse bards. Writing in elegant Icelandic prose, Snorri creates a fictional Swedish king, Gylfi, disguised as a beggar named Gangleri, who visits Asgard, the home of the gods (the Norse Olympus), to interview the also-disguised Odin (Wotan in Germany) and other figures about their history. This history is dark, but it reflects a process of cosmic birth, death and rebirth that will be familiar, for instance, to readers of the mythology of India. And, as in the mythology of India, sex plays a major role in Norse mythology.

The *Poetic Edda* and *Prose Edda* tell of two races of gods, the Vanir and the Aesir. The Vanir were fertility gods, closer to the earth and its productivity than the more distant warrior gods of Asgard led by Odin. Goddesses and sexuality – perhaps even orgies – were important to the early worshippers of the Vanir. Three of the most important deities of the Vanir were the sea god Njord and his children, the fertility god Freyr, and his equally fertile sister Freya. Freyr was typically depicted with an erection to illustrate his primary function. The Vanir were an expression of sexuality without moral boundaries. Incest, for instance, was freely practised by them; Njord's wife was also his sister. There is no sense here of love relating to sex – only lust that needs to be satisfied to keep the world fertile.

After a Norse version of the war in Heaven between the Vanir and Aesir, the two divine races became one or at least achieved a truce in which the fertility and warrior modes they represented were blended. But even when tied to the Aesir, the Vanir's role in the Norse cultural dream remained an expression of sexual lust combined with a willingness to use sex as a method of payment for the objects of other lusts. Two tales – one involving Freyr and one his sister Freya – are examples of Vanir sexuality.

The first myth is that of Freyr and the beautiful giantess Gerd, whose name means 'earth'. It is a myth, as Christopher Fee has suggested in *Gods, Heroes and Kings: The Battle for Mythic Britain* that 'runs the gamut of sexual and romantic imagery: lovesickness, reckless lust . . . phallic and vaginal symbolism, and references to Freyr's dominion over sexual fecundity.' The tale begins with a taboo. Freyr steals into Odin's sacred seat in Asgard, spies on the giantess in faraway Jotunheim and is immediately overcome by desire. Knowing the gods will never accept his union with the giant, Freyr falls into despair until finally his servant Skirnir agrees to visit Gerd to plead his master's case. But he agrees to do so only in return for several valuable gifts, including Freyr's magic sword that could fight under its own power. Here Freyr assumes the role of so many lovers in literary and actual history who sacrifice their own and their families' welfare for lust. By giving up his sword, Freyr metaphorically castrates himself. At Ragnarok, the end of the world, he will have no defence against the fire that will consume not only him but all fertility.

Arriving at Gerd's home, in a 'bowl-shaped dale covered with dismal gray grass', Skirnir is almost overcome by the cold there, but he approaches the giantess. After failing to convince her with various gifts, Skirnir waves a magic staff before her and threatens her with a curse that will leave her barren, untouchable and burdened with a hopeless, unconsummated and devouring lust. Gerd agrees to meet Freyr in nine days – a length of time that seems to Freyr like an eternity.

The Freyr–Gerd myth is parallel to one involving Freyr's father, Njord, and the giantess Skadi. In both cases, as Fee points out, the giantesses, representing cold earth, are fertilized by the 'life-giving force' that is the seed of the Vanir gods.

The second myth is that of the necklace of the Brisings. Two gods join Freya as the main characters in this story. They are the All Father Odin and the trickster Loki. Followed stealthily by Loki, Freya makes her way inside the mountain smithy of four dwarves. She has come there in search of jewels, and when she sees the spectacular Necklace of the Brisings she immediately desires it with all

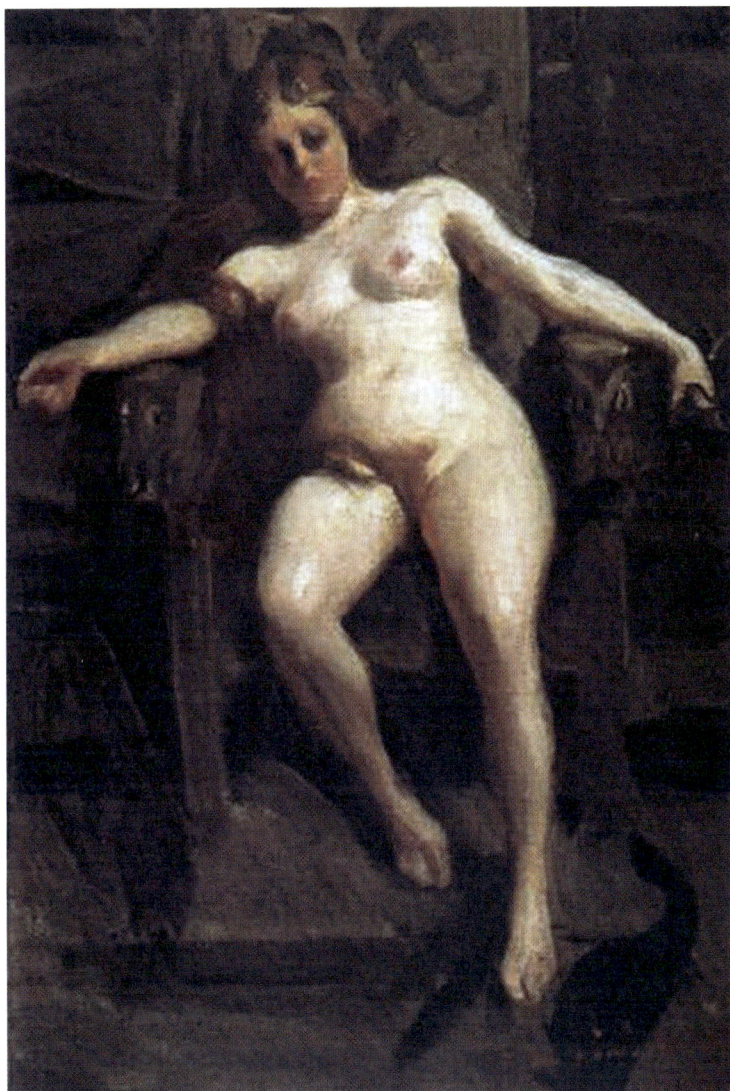

Anders Zorn, *Freya*, 1901, oil on canvas.

her being. The four dwarves are equally affected by the beauty of the goddess. Freya desires the necklace; the dwarves desire Freya. After much haggling, the dwarves demand the use of Freya's body and Freya agrees. After satisfying the dwarves in turn, Freya returns to Asgard, but is always followed by Loki who, while the goddess sleeps, steals her hard-earned necklace. Loki then goes to the All Father, gives him the necklace and reports what Freya has done to win it. Odin has for some time lusted after Freya himself and he is enraged by her having sex with the dwarves. Freya had become close to Odin, teaching him the *seidr*, the female magic of fecundity. That fertility magic is used by Odin with numerous partners. Freya was sometimes conflated with Frigg, the wife of Odin and daughter of Fjorgyn, whose name means 'earth'. Fjorgyn was also the mother of the great thunder god Thor, by her son-in-law, Odin himself, earth being the proper depository of the seed of the greatest of the Aesir.

In the case of the Brisings myth, Freya gets her necklace back – a necklace being a common Indo-European symbol of the Great Goddess – but only after she agrees to bring war and death to the human world of Midgard. Again, the myth reminds us that lust has a price, a price, however, that is of no importance to the Vanir.

One of the most sexual of the Norse gods was Loki. Tricksters, sometimes comic, sometimes dangerous characters, are nearly always associated with shape-shifting capabilities and with unbridled sexual appetites. They are always amoral. Loki is no exception. Often his sexually based tricks are of a puerile sort, as in the myth of Skadi's laugh. The gods have agreed with the giantess Skadi that she will not accept marriage with one of the Aesir unless one of them can make her laugh as she has never laughed before. Odin calls on Loki to achieve this goal. So, the trickster relates the story of an adventure he has recently had with a goat. He says he had tied one end of a thong to the goat's beard and the other end to his own testicles. He had then made a loud noise causing the goat to run forward. A tugging struggle ensued between the goat's beard and Loki's testicles. The coarse little story causes the giantess to laugh as she has never laughed before.

There is one story of Loki as a transsexual involved in an act of bestiality. The gods found themselves in a difficult position vis-à-vis the mason who was repairing the walls of Asgard assisted by a mighty stallion after the Vanir-Aesir war. Loki was called on to delay the mason's work to allow the gods to avoid making a payment they had agreed upon. To cause the delay Loki turned himself into a mare to attract the mason's stallion and the two horses galloped into the woods where the stallion had sex with the mare – really with Loki, who thus took the passive role (*ergi*) in a sex act, which in Norse tradition would be as looked down upon as it was in Greece and Rome and other societies of the world. Nevertheless, Loki was a trickster and socially deviant behaviour on his part was expected and could be excused. Excused or not, Loki turned up at Asgard some months later with a magic eight-legged colt named Sleipnir, the offspring of his tryst with the stallion.

Thor, the thunder god who rivals Odin as the most powerful of the Norse gods, was also involved in a gender reversal. When Thor woke one day to discover that his famous hammer, Mjollnir, was missing, he went to Loki for help. The two gods found that it was the giant Thrym who had stolen the hammer and hidden it deep in the earth, a sexual metaphor given the phallic nature of Thor's hammer (the hammer, for instance, was traditionally placed in the bride's lap in Viking marriage rites). The giant agreed to return the hammer only in return for marriage to the goddess Freya. When the gods informed Freya of the potential bargain she refused, and

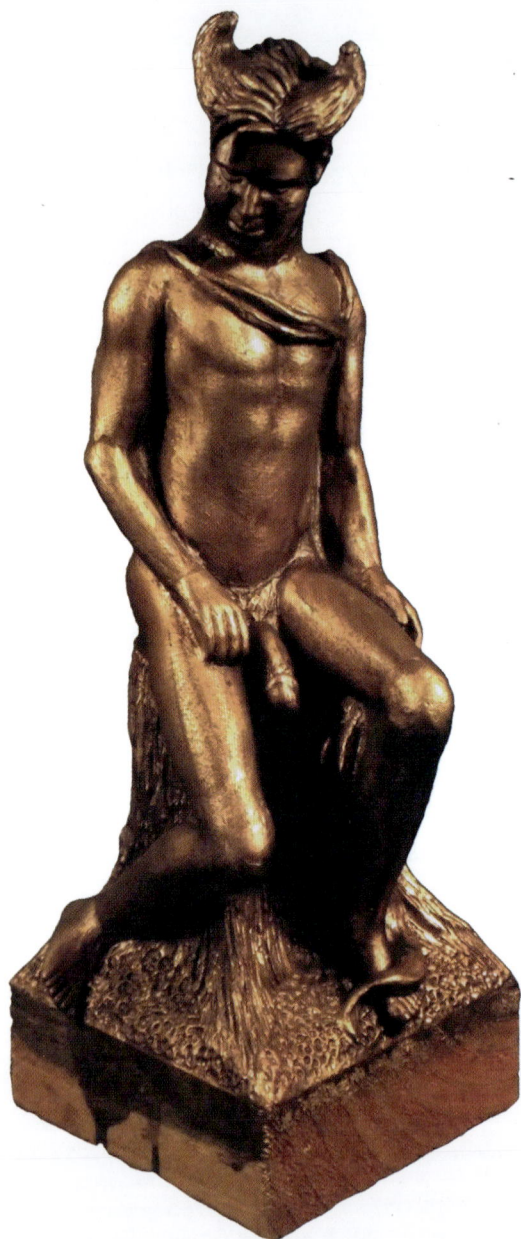

Malcolm Lidbury, *Loki*, 2015, bronze sculpture.

it was decided that Thor should disguise himself as the 'bride'. Humiliated by this undermining of his masculinity, Thor nevertheless agreed: anything to get back his hammer – his source of power, his manhood. He dressed as a beautiful young maiden with keys at his waist and the Necklace of the Brisings around his neck. The gods all teased the Thunderer for this *ergi* situation in which he found himself. Loki joined Thor, dressed as a bridesmaid. When the pair reached Thrym's home in Jotunheim, Thor (as Freya) sat at the waiting banquet table and, much to his (her) groom's surprise, devoured a whole roasted ox and several beakers of mead. The bridesmaid explained the bride's appetite as being the result of several days without food and a burning desire for the marriage bed. Thrym became so excited that he called for Thor's hammer to be placed on his bride's lap immediately so that he might achieve the goal of his lust. The moment the hammer was placed on Thor's lap he grasped it, revealed his identity, and with the return of his masculine power, threw off the female clothes and killed Thrym and the other giants at the wedding.

Celtic and Norse mythologies existed contemporaneously, and there are similarities. Both, except for the Arthurian tales and the Irish heroic ones, are concerned very little with ordinary human beings. It is the gods (and heroes) with whom they are preoccupied, as is the case with Mesopotamian, Egyptian and Indian mythologies. A very human experience, sex, plays a role in Celtic and Norse mythologies, but it is sex that centres around the gods. In the case of Irish mythology, the sex is even further removed as it is mostly sanitized by the monks who retold the tales. In the case of the Norse myths the sex is more explicit because the redactors, although Christian, had no interest in using the myths to express Christian values. The tales were, after all, only about deities who never really existed and whose sexuality was revealed either for humour – as was also the case with much of Greek mythology – or to speak to certain human tendencies. What the two Northern European traditions do have in common is the metaphorical use of myth to express a human struggle between unbridled desire and a necessary ordering of such desire into proper controlled ritualistic patterns. Thus, we have the Firbolg and Fomarian barbarism versus the sacred marriages between Celtic kings and their queens representing Sovereignty, and the unbridled sexuality of the fertility-driven ancient Vanir versus the social mores of the Aesir, mores which were themselves close to those of the Vikings who created these gods.

Seven

China and Japan

C HINESE AND JAPANESE mythologies both tend to de-emphasize
sex but contain elements that suggest its importance in versions
of myths that preceded the emergence of dominant Confucianism
in China and Buddhism in both places.

Chinese Mythology

Paintings on walls, shells and bones and even a structure apparently
dedicated to a goddess, suggests the existence of a prehistoric mythological system in the Neolithic Hongshan culture of northeast China
dating from the period between 4700 and 2900 BCE. By about 1400
BCE, during the Shang Dynasty, the earliest form of Chinese writing
had taken form and is generally known as the Oracle Bone Script
as it was apparently used in divination processes and was found on
tortoise shells and animal bones.

The fully written sources for Chinese mythology consist of
several collections. The most important, the *Shanhaijing* (Classic of
Mountains and Seas), although traditionally attributed to the mythical Emperor Yu, was composed gradually beginning in the fourth
century BCE under the Zhou Dynasty, its final version completed
during the Han Dynasty sometime between 206 BCE and 9 CE.

Another source, the *Chuci* (Poetry of the South), was compiled between 340 and 278 BCE. A third source, the *Huainanzi* (Masters of Huainan) was compiled in the middle of the second century BCE. The Chinese have tended, under the influence of secular Confucianism, to blend the so-called mythological period into what is considered actual history. That is, Confucian scholars were primarily concerned with ethics and proper government and preferred to see the ancient myths as metaphors and symbols that could be applied to real life. As a result, it is sometimes difficult to differentiate the imaginary people and events of the mythological period from those of actual Chinese history. The problem becomes more complex given the fact that there are myths from the many ethnic groups of China, groups with various mythological traditions. Furthermore, if Confucius (551–479 BCE) and his followers preferred to historicize the old myths, the other two primary Chinese religious and philosophical traditions, Taoism founded by Laozi (Lao-tse) (604–531 BCE) and Buddhism, introduced in about 150 BCE, had myths of their own or saw the myths from a different perspective from those who had originally told them in the prehistoric period. Taoists especially tended to interpret and reform myths to fit their own unique philosophy, so much so that the *Shanhaijing*, the *Chuci* and the *Huainanzi* can reasonably be called Taoist texts.

For many Chinese, the supreme Chinese deity was the Jade Emperor (Yudi), a Taoist version of an older Supreme Being, Tian Di or Shang Di. In the Chinese mytho-historical versions there were also the Three Sovereigns (Three August Ones) and the Five Emperors. Depending on the source, the Three Sovereigns are Fuxi, Nuwa and Shennong, and the emperors are Huangdi (the Yellow Emperor), Zuanxu (Gaoyang), Ku, Yao and Shun. Yao, Shun and Shun's successor Yu are called the Three Sage Kings. Yu was the founder of the Xia Dynasty, which preceded the historical Shang Dynasty. Sex plays a relatively minor role among these ancient deities. For the most part, the gods were treated as culture heroes who taught humans how to live and who dealt with calamities such as the great flood. Most were themselves miraculously conceived without the help of sex. In what are known as Gansheng myths, the mothers of gods and heroes conceived and/or were born in various ways, by eating certain plants, for instance, drinking certain fluids, or being exposed to the sun. Huangdi, the Yellow Emperor, was conceived by his mother Fubao by means of a bolt of lightning; Yu was born out of his father's corpse; Jiandi conceived her son Qi, the founder of the Shang Dynasty, after eating a swallow's nest. It might be that such myths have their origins in prehistoric times before the connection between intercourse and conception was understood. The *Shanhaijing* does occasionally tell of heroes being conceived via intercourse, but even then the conception is miraculous, as when a dragon copulates with a woman and conceives heroes such as the Yellow Emperor, Shennon and Shun, who then embody the great dragon's powers.

For some Chinese, the universe itself was created because of a miraculous birth. There are various versions of the myth, but they all begin with a cosmic egg in pre-creation Chaos. One myth tells how the egg contained a creator known as Pangu who, within the egg or by breaking out of the egg, separated the white from the yolk, thus creating Heaven and Earth, masculine Yang and feminine Yin.

The separation was gradual. Over 18,000 years Pangu grew taller and taller, pushing the two worlds apart. According to some versions, Pangu died eventually and his body parts became mountains, metals, rocks, streams and other elements of creation. His semen became pearls. This animistic approach to creation is reminiscent of the Mesopotamian myth of Marduk creating the world from the dead body of the great mother, Tiamat, and of similar stories in Native American myths.

The Pangu myth is a version of the Earth and Sky separation theme shared with mythologies from many cultures. In another Chinese separation myth, the deities Zhong and Li are instructed by the high god to separate Earth and Sky, so as to punish the people by making it impossible for them to ascend to Heaven. In a somewhat scatological version, the people on Earth eat too much and produce so much excrement that the supreme being raises Heaven away from Earth to avoid the unpleasant odour. The Chinese separation myths are less explicitly sexual than those of Mesopotamia, Egypt, Oceania, Greece and elsewhere, where Heaven and Earth are locked in constant sexual intercourse, making further creation impossible and causing a relative of the first parents to separate them, sometimes violently. It seems likely that originally a similar Chinese myth existed. One version of the Zhong and Li separation implies this when we are told that there was no room between Heaven and Earth to stand up. In general, however, the extant versions of the myth have almost certainly been sanitized by Taoist and Confucian views.

A Vietnamese version of the Sky-Earth myth before the separation contains a glimpse into what the Chinese myth might once have looked like. Vietnamese mythology borrows heavily from Chinese traditions. The myth in question is overtly sexual. It tells how a giant was at work creating the world when a female appeared. The two developed a highly amorous relationship but fought often, too. The female was the stronger of the two and she had a much larger sex organ. These figures are representations of Heaven and Earth. After a time, during which they vied with each other over creative ability, the giant and the woman decided to marry. On the way to his bride's house the groom and his hundred attendants were blocked by a river. Undeterred, the giant used his huge penis as a bridge and all went well until a spark landed on the penis, causing the giant to lurch so violently that half his companions fell off. These were rescued by the woman, who put them under her dress to warm them up. The sex organs of both beings prove to be of equal value; together they form the wholeness which is Yin linked to Yang.

A popular Chinese myth about the creation of humans is somewhat sexual in nature. Like several Indian creation myths it involves the incestuous relationship between a brother and a sister, who are the only beings alive after a great flood. Brother and sister are humans in some versions of the myth, but more often the pair are identified with the god Fuxi, who represents the warmth of Yang, and the goddess Nuwa, who is Yin. The two ask the Jade Emperor for and receive a sign allowing them to copulate incestuously to repopulate the world.

The category seemingly little affected by Confucian conservatism is folklore in the provinces, especially in the south. Here sex is a common theme. In his *Asian Mythologies* Yves Bonnefoy points out, for instance, that Fubao's conception of the Yellow Emperor takes place in 'an uncultivated countryside (*ye*)', suggesting the sort of sacred fertility place where young peasants form 'irregular unions . . . at the time of agricultural festivals'. Bonnefoy also discusses southern love songs that were condemned for their licentiousness by the Confucian authorities. In one such song Yu comes down from the sky to have intercourse with the woman who will be his wife. Their rendezvous takes place in the 'Mulberry Trees of the Terrace', a probable allusion to Mulberry Forest, traditionally 'the land of song' in which gatherings of boys and girls took place in what were, in effect, 'sexual festivals'.

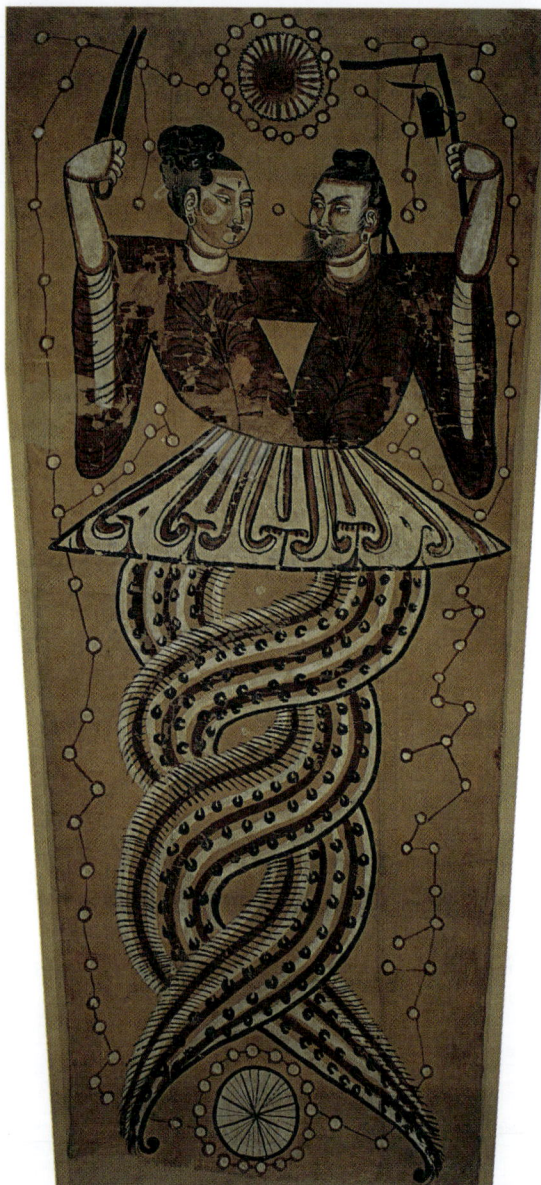

Nuwa and Fuxi, Xinjiang,
possibly 3rd century CE, hanging silk scroll.

There are several deities specifically associated with sex. A goddess, Jiutian Xuannu, resembles the many goddesses of the Middle East and Europe who are associated both with love and war. She is particularly known for teaching the arts of sex, as contained in such works as *The Mysterious Woman Classic* and *The Natural Woman Classic* during the Han Dynasty, and in the seventh-century CE *The Bedchamber Arts of the Master of the Grotto Mysteries*, all containing explicit descriptions of sex acts. Works like these are clearly influenced by a Taoist concept of 'chi' (life energy), which is associated with the sex act. In this context intercourse was a spiritual exercise in which such practices as avoiding ejaculation serve to preserve chi. The joining of man and woman was a joining of Heaven (Yang) and Earth (Yin). The original Taoist view sees a process in which the woman plays an equal role with the man. The Confucian position on the superiority of the male has tended to overcome that view.

Tu Er Shen (rabbit god) is a deity who protects homosexuals. It is said that he was once a man named Hu Tianbao who desired a handsome young imperial officer and was caught spying on him. Hu Tianbao confessed his 'sin' and was executed. But the lords of the underworld forgave this crime of love and made Hu Tianbao the homosexual god Tu Er Shen.

Homosexuality is a common theme in Chinese folk traditions, and in some provinces man-boy love, much as practised in Greece, was acceptable. There are many stories of *Xian* (animal spirits) having homosexual relationships with men. The dragon, a symbol of male sexual power, is attracted to men in some myths. There is the story, for instance, of the farmer who is sodomized by a dragon. Other homoerotic farmer stories include pig and fox spirits.

Overall, however, in Chinese mythology sex plays a relatively minor role. The canonical mythology has been transformed in many cases into pseudo-history by the Confucians in an effort to avoid the supernatural. As for Buddhists, celibacy was a principle value. Myths for Confucians are used primarily as object lessons to support ethical and patriarchal principles. The Taoists have been more accepting of the mythical stories themselves, with all their supernatural aspects, including miraculous births and especially regarding the Three August Ones and the Five Emperors. For Taoists, the events described in the great mythological texts serve as philosophical vehicles leading the reader to Taoist values. For Taoists, sex is an important way of expressing those values, and it is reasonable to suppose that the ancient Taoist myths, as indicated by local folklore, expressed this fact before giving way to the patriarchal views of the Confucians.

Japanese Mythology

Sex plays a significant role in Shinto, the way of the gods (kami). The origins of this indigenous religion can be traced back to the hunter-gathering people of the Jomon culture, who inhabited Japan from perhaps as early as *c.* 14,000 BCE. Archaeologists of the Jomon period have uncovered small statues (*dogu*) of women, many pregnant, statues not unlike the 'Venuses' of Neolithic Europe and Asia Minor, and phallic-suggesting stone cylinders (*sekibo*) such as those found in the Indus Valley, Ireland and elsewhere.

These articles have been associated by scholars with fertility and phallic cults. Fertility, phallicism and authority – especially male authority – are all aspects of Shinto as it developed. The first literary records of Shinto, or proto-Shinto, are found in the *Weishi*, chronicles of the Chinese Wei Dynasty of the third century. These chronicles tell of a shaman queen, Himiko, who was likely one of many such queens, and who had great powers as a ruler. Himiko perhaps represented an early matriarchal aspect in Japan, one that was somewhat preserved in more formalized Shinto by the great sun goddess Amaterasu. Shinto, however, became clearly patriarchal, as indicated by the myths contained in the two major Japanese mythological texts, the *Kojiki* (Record of Ancient Matters), completed in 712 CE, and the *Nihongi* (Chronicles of Japan), completed in 720 CE. These sacred books of Shinto contain myths based on much earlier versions formerly transmitted orally. Their primary figures are the creators of Japan, Izanagi and his sister-wife Izanami, and Amaterasu and her brother Susanowo.

In the beginning, as in most mythologies, Heaven and Earth existed together in a chaotic mix. Then somehow a separation took place as light particles rose to form a distinct Heaven (Yo or Yang) and heavier ones stayed below and became Earth (In or Yo). Creation was now possible. Five genderless gods emerged from Heaven, followed by two more. Finally, five pairs of gendered gods appeared. The last of these were Izanagi and his sister Izanami. It was they who were designated by the older gods to create the world, which is to say, in the context of Shinto, Japan.

Izanagi (he who invites) and Izanami (she who invites) were given a jewelled spear (*Ame-no-nuboko*) and, standing on the floating Bridge of Heaven, they used the spear to stir up the undefined mass below until a salty substance come out of the tip of the instrument and formed the first Japanese island. The creator couple then came down and built a central column (*Ame-no-mihashira*) to complete the separation of Heaven and Earth.

The next step was procreation. As in so many mythologies, original procreation would depend upon the incestuous relationship between a brother and sister. It begins with a bodily examination.

Izanagi asks his sister about her body and she answers that it is fully formed except for one part which has not grown. Izanagi notes that his body, too, is fully formed but for one part which has grown excessively. He suggests that he use that part to fill up the part of his sister's anatomy which is less grown. In this way, he says, they will create more things and places. Izanami agrees, and Izanagi proposes a ritual in which they will move in opposite directions around the world pillar until they meet, at which time they will have sexual intercourse.

When they did meet during the ritual, Izanami spoke first: 'What a fine youth you are,' she said. Izanagi answered in kind but then criticized Izanami for speaking first: 'A wife should never speak first,' he cried. Nevertheless, they had intercourse and the result was two badly formed children. This, said the old gods, was the fault of the woman, who had spoken first.

The couple returned to the pillar and repeated their ritual circumambulation, and this time Izanagi spoke first before they had intercourse. The result was more Japanese islands. Izanami's genitals were destroyed and she died giving birth to fire. After she went to the underworld Izanagi attempted to retrieve her but failed. When he returned to the world Izanagi and Izanami's most famous offspring, Amaterasu, was born from her father's left eye. Izanagi appointed his daughter to the rulership of the sky. Amaterasu had a younger brother, Susanowo (the Impetuous Male), a storm god with whom, as the sun, she constantly quarrelled.

Theirs was a war between light and darkness, and, it must be said, between male and female. In one conflict, which would surely have interested Freud, Amaterasu seizes her brother's sword and bites it into pieces, thus forming three goddesses. After a particularly despicable act of drunkenness on the part of her brother, the Great

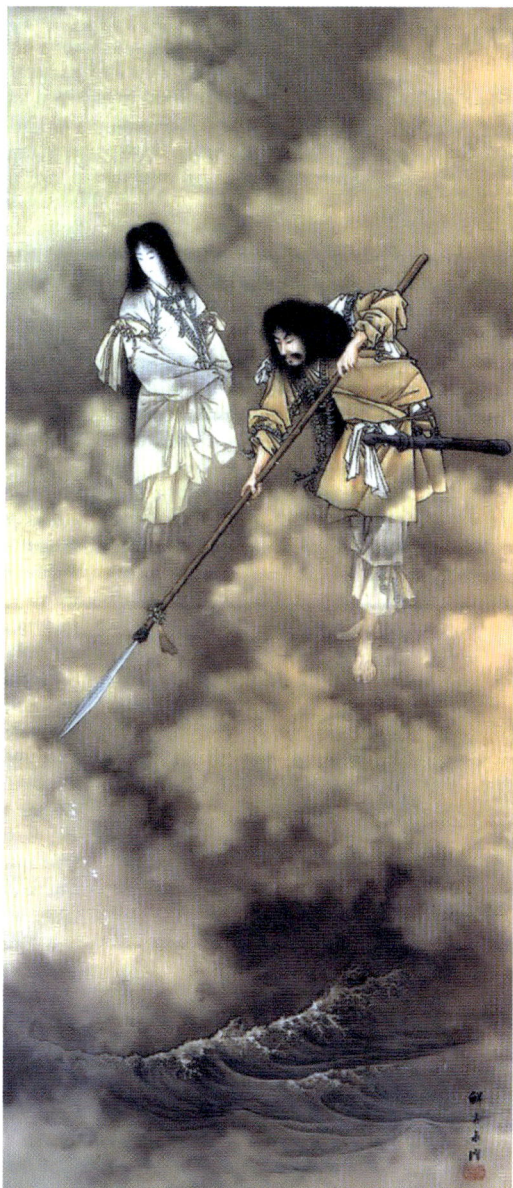

Kobayashi Eitaku, *Izanagi and Izanami Creating
the Japanese Islands*, 1885, hanging silk scroll.

Goddess retreats to her cave and locks herself in, thus depriving the world of light and warmth. In so doing Amaterasu follows in the footsteps of the Hittite god Telipinu, who disappeared and left the world barren, and the Greek Demeter, who deprived the world of fertility when her daughter Persephone was raped. In the case of Amaterasu, she is lured back by a highly sexual dance performed in front of the cave by the goddess Ame no Uzume. The dance myth is very likely the source of Shinto rituals held in winter to bring about the renewal in spring of the sun's power.

In both the Izanagi–Izanami and Amaterasu–Susanowo myths the question of proper relationships between males and females – in both domestic and cosmic senses – is paramount. Although Amaterasu is said to be the ancestress of emperors in the land of her rising sun, the message of the Izanagi–Izanami myth is clearly reflective of the tradition of male dominance in Japanese society. Their acts suggest proper roles of the male and female in the sex act as well as in the larger creative process. The male's role is to speak and act first, to fill the gap which defines the female with the part that defines him as a male. Izanami undermines the quest for male–female union and cosmic order by speaking first in the couple's initial attempt to procreate. Only when Izanagi speaks first can procreation proceed properly.

In terms of creation itself the same principle applies. Izanami stands by Izanagi on the bridge of Heaven and they wield the phallic spear given them by the old gods. The fluid that drips from the spear in the formless amniotic mass below creates Japan – the world. In this way, separated Heaven and Earth are spiritually reunited. This is what the Chinese would call a Yang act. When the couple circumambulate the also phallic world pillar the second time, they are performing a Yin act and in so doing they properly complete the Yin-Yang unity. Izanagi is the primordial Yang, Izanami the primordial Yin.

That being said, the myth of Izanami's death and the failure of Izanagi to retrieve her culminates in enmity between the two. It is Izanami who disappears from view and Izanagi who continues the creative process culminating in Amaterasu, who exists in a world dominated not by the 'part not grown' but by the 'part grown excessively'. The world that Izanagi leaves behind when he retires from the scene is a phallocentric one.

The Shinto pantheon of popular belief contains phallic gods, and related festivals and shrines. Shinto brides were often given sex manuals called *shunga* (spring pictures) containing explicit illustrations of 'proper' sexual positions, usually featuring phalli of extreme proportions.

Once considered useful in warding off infertility or other problems, phallic shrines – like the Greek Herms – were set up at strategic

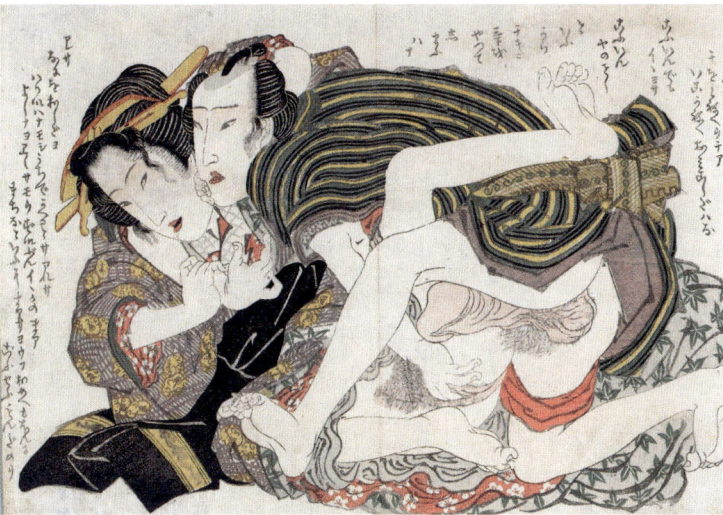

Keisai Eisen, *Green Shirt*, 1825, *shunga*.

places in villages. Although discouraged now, women would decorate these shrines in hopes of achieving wishes.

Phallic festivals still exist in Japan. Perhaps the most famous is the Kanamara Matsuri, the 'Steel Penis Festival', held annually at the Kanayama shrine in Kawasaki. Celebrators at the festival watch a parade featuring a phallus of huge proportions, and are treated to such delicacies as candy and vegetable phalli.

The basis of the Kanamara Matsuri is a myth involving a demon that hid in a vagina and bit off the penises of young men. The demon was de-fanged when a blacksmith created a steel penis which succeeded in breaking the demon's teeth. This is a version of the vagina

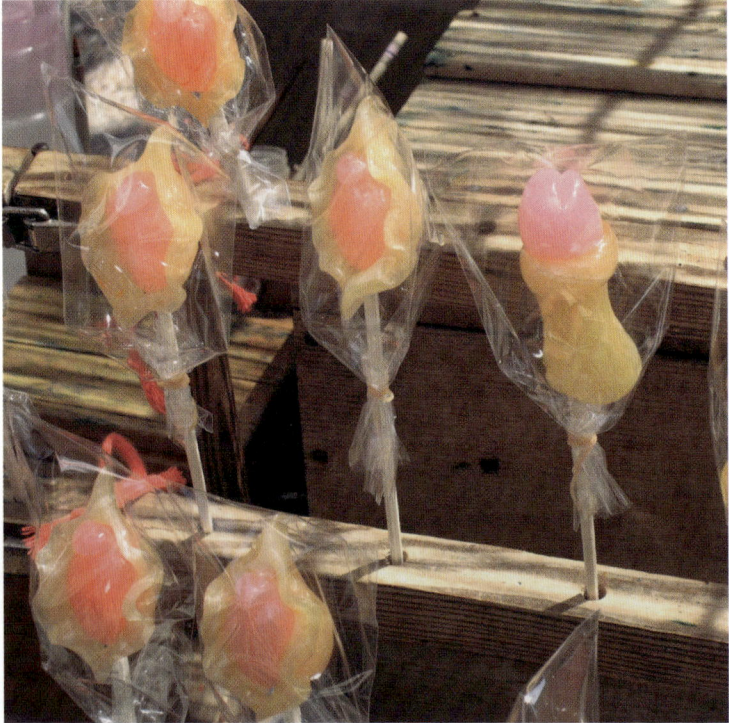

Penis candies made for the Kanamara Matsuri festival.

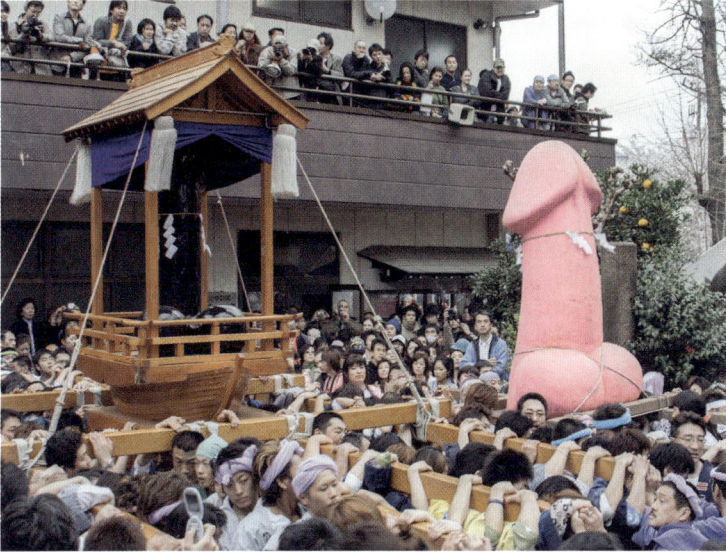

Metal phallus made for the Kanamara Matsuri festival.

dentata myth which exists in many parts of the world, including, for instance, in Native North America and Polynesia.

Homosexuality exists in Shinto mythology. Shinu No Hafuri and Ama No Hafuri were male servants of the goddess Amaterasu and were deeply in love. When Shinu died, Ama committed suicide to be with his lover forever. A homosexual tradition involving *wakushū*, adolescent boys, a 'third gender' available to both men and women, led to a type of Japanese print celebrating the beauty of these boys and, by implication, the superiority or at least comparability of sex with them over love between adult males and females. This tradition, called *shudo*, resembles similar ones in China, Egypt, Greece, Rome and elsewhere. In the seventeenth-century *The Great Mirror of Male Love*, the author, Ihara Saikaku, wrote: 'It is sacrilege to speak of female love in the same breath as boy love . . . a youth is like the first plum blossom of the new year.'

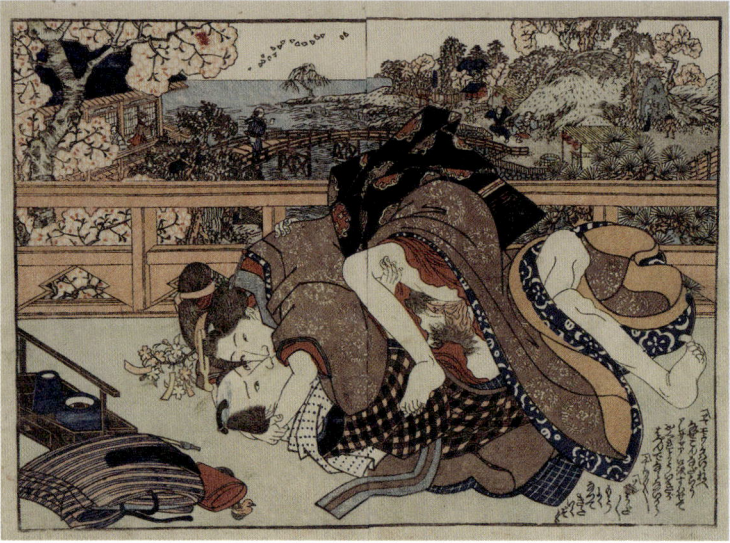

Man with *wakushū*, c. 1790, *shunga*.

To summarize, sex is not as evident in Chinese or Japanese mythology as it is, for instance, in Greek or Indian mythology. To the extent that it does exist it seems to serve as a means of establishing a view of social structure in which masculine, patriarchal values are dominant but in which there is a longing for union between male and female Yang and Yin – to achieve cosmic order.

Eight

Sub-Saharan Africa

AFRICA IS A CONTINENT of multiple cultures and mythologies. Some of these mythologies reach back to the origins of Homo sapiens; others have been 'corrupted' by later influences. The Efe people of the Democratic Republic of the Congo, for instance, tell a story of the origins of humans and sin that clearly reflects the influence of Christian missionaries. According to this Adam and Eve myth, the creator, Baatsi, made humans – male and female – out of clay and commanded them to procreate. Their only restriction was to not eat of the Tahu Tree. At some point a female descendant of the first couple convinced her husband to break off fruit from the tree and together they ate it. The result was the institution of death for humans.

When not overly influenced by the perspectives of the organized religions of conquerors and colonists – religions such as Islam and Christianity – African myths are essentially animistic. Animism can reasonably be assumed to be the oldest of religions. It is the religion of peoples who see a spiritual animation in all aspects of the material world. The myths of animism tell of interactions between humans and the spirits among whom they live.

Often African myths centre on creator deities who are the source of the animation. Earth goddesses are sometimes important, as are tricksters and culture heroes, those figures who either interfere with creation or teach the people how to survive in it. Many themes present in other mythologies are also found in African mythologies, including creative incest, often experienced by sacred twins; the separation of Heaven and Earth; intimate contact between gods and humans; and the erotic exploits of tricksters.

Creation stories are basic to all cultures and it is not surprising that Africans, like people in other parts of the world, use the process of procreation as an appropriate metaphor for the creation of the world. In patriarchal cultures, such as many of those in Africa, creation can come directly from the semen of the male creator, as it does in the Egyptian creation by masturbation, for instance. One ancient sub-Saharan rock painting reveals such a creator, reclining on his side as semen leaves his penis and animates all the elements of life.

A particularly important theme in African mythologies is that of the separation of Heaven and Earth. This separation as treated

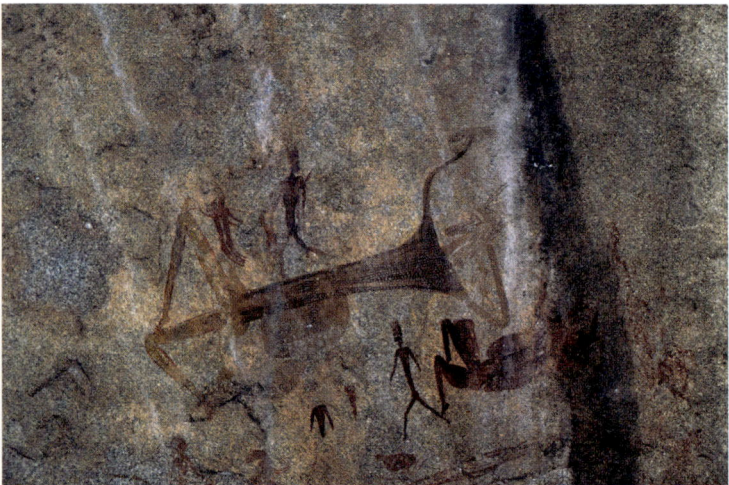

A scene from the 'Diana's Vow' rock paintings, showing the Creator ejaculating creation, Zimbabwe Eastern Highlands, *c*. 5000 BCE.

in Africa is often associated with the *deus absconditus* or *deus otiosus* (the god who disappears or abandons) archetype. The Bushmen (San) who live in the Kalahari Desert of Botswana and South Africa say their creator, Mantis, whose daughter married a snake, lived on Earth, taking many animal forms, but that he became disgusted with humans and left. In this case the god, for various reasons, decides to abandon humanity, and, by extension, Earth itself, to its own devices without his further participation.

The Krachi people of Togo and Ghana tell another kind of separation story, one that is mythologically closely linked to similar stories in Egypt, Greece and many other parts of the world. In the beginning, there was the god Wulbari (Heaven), who was in constant conjunction with the goddess Asase Ya (Earth). The couple created men and women who lived between them and mated with each other. But the people had little room to move easily, and their squirming irritated Wulbari. He was particularly bothered by an old woman who kept hitting him with her pestle as she ground her maize, and by another woman who cut off bits of him to spice up her soup. Finally, Wulbari became so fed up that he lifted himself from Asase Ya and remained far above her out of reach. The people were now free to move about, but, as in so many myths, without the god's presence they became vulnerable to problems – particularly to death.

Some Dinka of Sudan have a first couple myth of separation that may have been slightly influenced by the Book of Genesis but which is essentially indigenous. The creator Nhialic, they say, created the first humans by moulding clay figures and placing them in pots. Out of one pot the first male, Garang, emerged with a fully-formed 'spear' or penis. The first female, Abuk, sprang from her pot with breasts and proper genitals. The creator ordered the pair to mate and announced that their progeny would die, but only for fifteen days. Garang objected to this reality, arguing that limiting death in this way would result in too large a population to feed. Abuk broke another divine command by planting more seeds than the creator had instructed her to plant. Nhialic grew so angry at this human independence that he cut the rope that tied Heaven to Earth and departed from the world as another example of the African *deus absconditus*.

African creation myths often involve explanations of the origins of sexuality. In a West African myth, told by the Ashanti people, the high god sent a Python spirit to teach the men and women he had created how to mate. As the men and women had no sexual urge, the Python had to devise a ritual (one still practised by some Ashanti) to create desire. He told the men and women to stand facing each other. He then took water from the river into his mouth and sprayed it on the fronts of their bodies. As he did so he said 'kus kus', words still used as part of a fertility ritual, and told them to go home and to face each other lying down. The men and women did as they were told and soon the women conceived.

The Wahungwe and Wakaranga of Zimbabwe have a myth which approaches the connection between the origins of sexuality and death and involves incest. In the beginning the creator, Maori, made the first man, Mwuetsi (the Moon), and placed him in the primeval waters. But Mwuetsi begged Maori to place him on Earth. The creator agreed but warned the man that living on Earth would involve the experience of death. When he got to Earth Mwuetsi found it to be barren and complained to the creator. The creator sent him a woman, Massassi (Morning Star), who brought fire with her. Maori said she could stay with Mwuetsi for two years. At night, the man and the woman lay on opposite sides of the fire. Mwuetsi began to wonder why Maori had sent the woman. On an impulse, he climbed over the fire and touched Massassi with his finger, which he had dipped in oil given him originally by the creator. Then he went back to his side of the fire and slept. In the morning Massassi was pregnant and soon gave birth to all the plants and trees of Earth. The couple lived together happily until the two years were up and Maori took Massassi away. Mwuetsi wept bitterly for several years until Maori sent another woman, Morongo (Evening Star), but again he said that the woman could stay for only two years. On their first night together, Mwuetsi leapt over the fire and touched Morongo with his oiled finger. But Morongo said that was not good enough. They would have to use the oil to lubricate their genitals, she said. And then they would have to have intercourse. Mwuetsi agreed and every night the couple had intercourse and every morning Morongo gave birth to the animals of the world and finally to human children. One night Maori sent a terrible storm to Earth and warned Mwuetsi that all his procreating would lead inevitably to death. He ordered the couple to stop having intercourse. Now Morongo became an Eve-like femme fatale. She had Mwuetsi close the door when they made love so Maori could not see them. And soon after that Morongo gave birth to violent animals – lions, leopards, snakes and the like. Now Morongo became more evil. She told Mwuetsi to have intercourse with his daughters. He did so and his children became the mothers of his people.

One night Morongo decided to couple with a snake. As is evident in many ancient mythologies, goddesses are frequently associated with snakes, snakes having a phallic aspect. When on another night Mwuetsi demanded that Morongo have sex with him she agreed, but during the act Morongo's snake-lover bit him and he became ill. As a result, his progeny, the plants and animals, began to die.

The people learned that only by sacrificing Mwuetsi and Morongo could fertility be restored. So they killed the couple and buried them together, and life returned to their progeny. The two years allowed by Maori had passed and he reminded the people that he had said that Mwuetsi's lovemaking and fertility would inevitably involve the experience of death.

Another story of the origins of sexuality is one told by the Dogon people of present-day Mali and Western Sudan. Dogon mythology is part of one of the most complex African religious systems. A Dogon cosmic egg creation myth involves sacred twins known as the Nummo (Nommo). In the beginning, there was only the creator Amma and the cosmic egg. A movement of the universe – some say the vibrations of the Digitaris seed – caused the maternal egg to break into two placental sacs, each housing a set of twins fertilized by Amma. In each sac one twin was male, one female, but each contained the essence of the other sex as well. These were the Nummo twins. Somehow a male twin, Yurugu, broke out of his placenta too early and a piece of his placental sac became the Earth. Yurugu tried to get back to his twin but she had left their sac and moved into the other sac with the other twins. So Yurugu, now alone, went back to the newly formed Earth, made from his own maternal placenta, and tried to copulate with it. As the copulation did not result in children, the creator sent the twins of the second sac and Yurugu's twin to Earth to copulate with each other – brothers, sisters and cousins. The result was humans.

In the context of Dogon marriage and kinship rituals and traditions, it would seem to be that since all humans are descended from either a mother and twin brother or a father and a twin sister, brothers and sisters can be parents of each other's children. According to some anthropologists, a Dogon man will, if possible, marry his first cousin by his maternal uncle after having sexual relations with his future mother-in-law or aunt. Given a basic incest taboo, this is as close as the man can come to intercourse with his mother – the ideal spouse in the Dogon mythological sense. Since the original twins contained the essence of the opposite sex and were, therefore, in a sense androgynous, Dogon children – male and female – had to be fully differentiated sexually by being circumcised, symbolizing the removal of the opposite sex from their bodies.

Another Dogon creation myth, as told by the Dogon sage Ogotommeli to the French ethnologist Marcel Griaule, is more overtly sexual and had the purpose of validating female circumcision. According to this myth, Amma created the Earth by throwing a piece of clay into space, the clay becoming a female figure lying horizontal, the head being to the north, the feet to the south, and the outstretched arms to the east and west. Earth's pubis took the form of an anthill and the clitoris was a termite hill. Amma was lonely and desired a female companion, but when he approached Earth, her clitoris rose in a male-like way and blocked his admission to her vagina. Amma solved the problem by cutting down the clitoris.

For some Dogon people Amma's rape of Earth resulted in the jackal, a symbol of all of Earth's problems. For others, the result was a version of the Nummo twins. In this case they were human from head to loins and serpents below. These Nummos contained the essence of Amma as well as of each other. Amma taught them what they needed to know about living in the world and by their transcending gender opposites they acted as an African Yin and Yang, bringing harmony to life.

Although African mythologies, including the Dogon, are generally patriarchal, featuring male creators, there are powerful goddesses who are sometimes creators as well. Among the Ibo of

Nigeria, the Earth Goddess Ala is such a figure. The West African Baga tribe worship Nimba, a similar figure. In both tribes women are valued more than in many others. In Dahomey there is the tradition of an androgynous head god named Mawu-Lisa; Mawu is the moon and Lisa the sun. Like other androgynous mythic figures, their union signifies the wholeness and balance of the good life and an ideal equality between men and women.

African myths, however, almost universally suggest the superiority of men over women. Sarah Dening points out in *The Mythology of Sex* that there are women's myths in Africa that tell of a time when women were once equal to men, only to lose that equality through the act of sex. A Masai myth from Kenya remembers a time when women were brave warriors. In those days women had no vaginas, only small urinary holes. They sometimes accompanied men, known as 'moran', into battle. On one such occasion these men came up behind the women in a campsite at night and pierced them between the legs with their 'spears', thus creating vaginas. After that, the men copulated with the women, whose lives became directed towards childbearing and serving men.

An important aspect of African mythologies – especially of West Africa – is the trickster. He can be, for example, the Yorubu Legba or Eshu or the Ashanti Anansi (the Spider). The African trickster, like his Native North American mythological brothers Cayote and Iktome, is amoral. Although he sometimes assists the creator, he more often does something to undermine creation itself. The point is, he pleases himself. He has immense appetites for the essentials of life such as food and sex. Ananse even steals his wife Aso from her father, the creator god. Psychologically the trickster is our childhood instincts unencumbered by what Freud called the superego. He can change shapes at will and he has no moral restraints. His

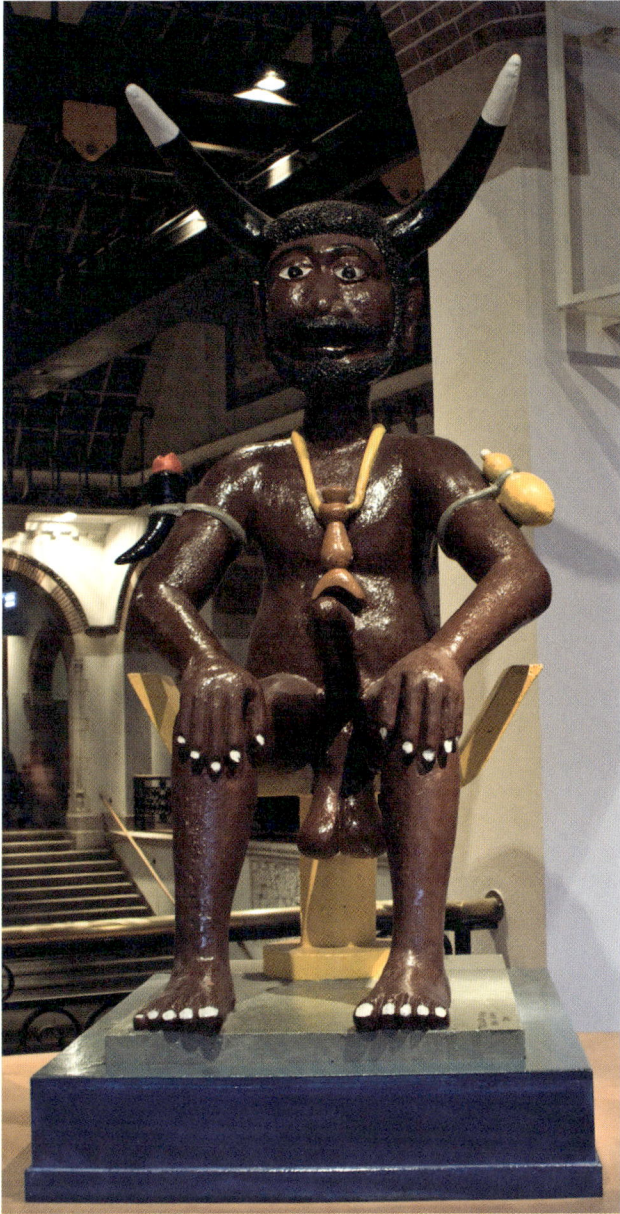

Ithyphallic Legba, date and artist unknown.

phallocentric depictions in tribal art emphasize his sexual appetite. Sometimes he is a household god, like the Greek Hermes (also a trickster) who also took phallocentric form in the household *herm*. When he wishes, the trickster can indulge in taboo acts such as homosexual ones. Whatever he does, he has no modesty. As a shape-shifter, he remains a sexual being.

The West African trickster came by way of the slave trade into the Americas, where he became figures such as Papa Legba in Haitian Voodoo and Aunt Nancy (for Ananse) among North American slaves.

As in the case of tricksters elsewhere, the trickster represents a fascination with sex, especially the male's fascination with his genitals, as well as a longing to transcend the established rules of conduct which can inhibit creativity.

Nine

Oceania

OCEANIA IS A vast area stretching from Australia and New Zealand all the way to Hawaii. The indigenous peoples of Oceania with the most complex mythologies are those of Australia and the Polynesian islands of the Pacific.

Australian Mythology

The indigenous Australians are commonly called Aboriginals. The ancestors of these people left Africa some 75,000 years ago, migrated into South Asia and then to Australia. The Aboriginals have been in Australia for at least 40,000 years, probably more, meaning that they can claim the longest connection with a particular land of any human group since the movement of Homo sapiens out of Africa. There are, of course, many Aboriginal tribes in Australia with various mythological traditions. What unifies these traditions is the concept of the Dreaming or Dreamtime and certain core figures and events, including the centrality of sex.

The Dreaming refers to a creation time when supernatural ancestors or spirit figures, acting as culture heroes, travelled across the continent in 'walkabouts' animating the world, creating forms of life and establishing people, animals and sacred places through

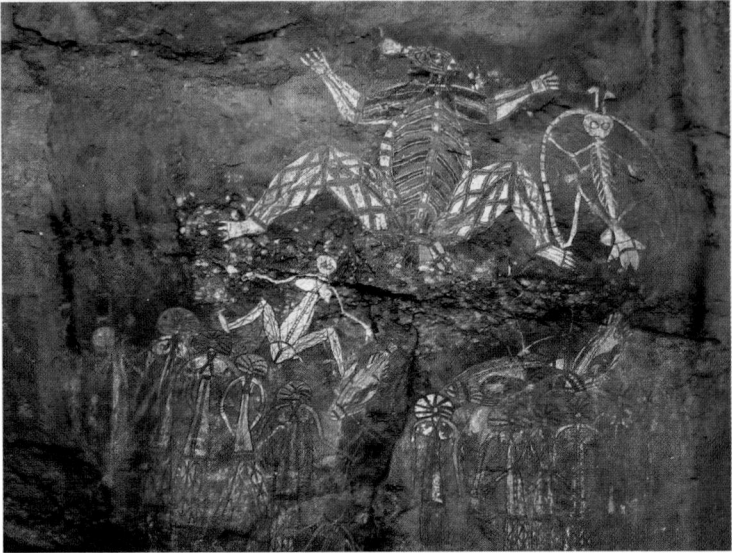

Rock art depicting Aboriginal ancestors, Kakadu National Park, *c.* 18,000 BCE.

their actions. Stories of the Dreamtime are thus myths of a group's
ancestry. Included in the Dreaming are several archetypal themes
familiar to readers of other mythologies. These include, for instance,
the birthing goddess and creative incest – archetypes with significant
sexual components.

In northern Australia the fertility Mother Goddess is Kunapipi.
She is Earth itself and her body contains the secret caves worshipped
by her followers. She is sometimes called 'the Old Woman' and is
associated, like many Great Goddesses of other cultures, with a serpent, in this case Ungud, the 'Rainbow Snake'. The snake opened
the way for Kunapipi as she walked about creating. The snake can
be seen as a symbol of the phallus and of the coital rites associated
with the goddess. These rites involve the moving up and down of a
phallic stick and erotic dancing simulating coitus, as well as actual
intercourse among the participants.

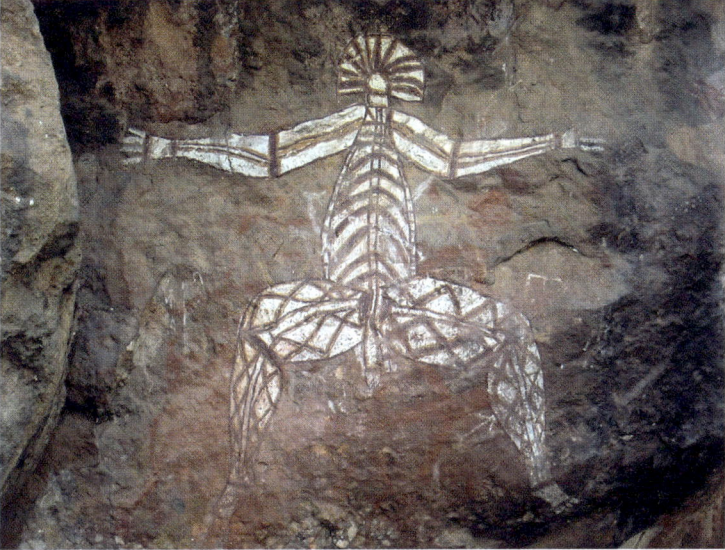

Aboriginal ancestors, Kakadu National Park, *c.* 18,000 BCE.

Some of the male participants have undergone subincision, in which an opening has been cut in the underside of the penis creating a vaginal-like entrance, the opening representing the Mother Goddess. In some cases ritual intercourse is performed in the subincision. For some the subincision is justified by the Rainbow Snake, who can be thought of as an andogynous creature with both male and female genitals. In the case of young girls, circumcision is common, as is the practice of introcision – a ritual stretching of the genitals – and the introduction of early intercourse.

One of the most popular of the Dreamtime creation myths is that of the Dhuwa group of the Yolngu people of northeastern Arnhem Land. They tell the myth in a song cycle meant to accompany fertility rituals. The story involves two sisters and a brother, collectively known as the Djanggawul. In the beginning these figures were the ancestors of human beings. The Djanggawul travelled about creating, using their sacred Dreamtime thoughts and various sacred objects that they carried with them in their bark canoe. The brother had a very long, uncircumcised, decorated penis. His sisters had long clitorises. The three siblings dragged their genitals along the ground wherever they went, leaving markings still sacred today.

Wherever the Djanggawul stopped, the brother had intercourse with one of his sisters. To do so it was necessary to raise their clitorises to clear a path for his penis. The result of these acts was human

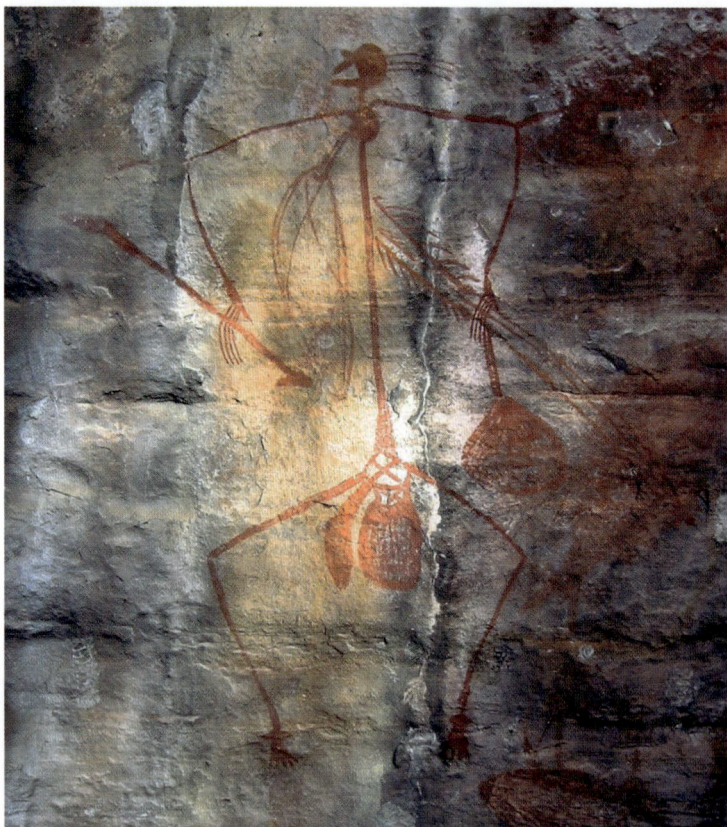

Aboriginal Kunapipi rite dancers, Kakadu National Park,
c. 18,000 BCE.

178

children. For these children, the Djanggawul left other Dreaming objects such as sacred stories and rites, still performed today. The sex organs of the Djanggawul are central to these myths and rituals and are represented by decorated phallic poles. The Djanggawul came to Jelangbara, now the centre of their cult, where they made a waterhole by thrusting one of these sacred poles into the ground. It is said by some that when they got to Jelangbara, to make their genitals less cumbersome they instituted male and female circumcision and perhaps introcision and subincision.

The importance of genitals – especially male genitals – in what is a generally patriarchal society is evident in Dreaming myths of the Kakadu people of northern Australia and of the Arandan people of central Australia along the Upper Fiske River. The Kakadu myth concerns the giant Wuraka, who walked about his world carrying his enormous penis over his shoulder. He met Imberombera – an equivalent of Kunapipi, and filled her with spirit children. In the Arandan myth the creator is Karora, who is identified with his phallic *tnatantja* pole, the source of his creative powers. In the beginning, Karora was sleeping under the rich soil and plants of Ilbalintja. There was only darkness in the world until a finely decorated *tnatantja* pole arose from the ground where the creator slept. The pole (like Shiva's lingam) reached all the way to the sky. The roots of the pole rested on the creator's head and he began to 'dream' creation, including the sun. The warmth of the sun caused Karora to burst out of the Earth, leaving the Ilbalintja Soak filled with the sweet juice of the honeysuckle, perhaps symbolic of the god's semen. The soak is there to this day.

Polynesian Mythology

The people known collectively as Polynesians began a migration to the Pacific as early as 3,500 years ago, probably from East Asia, using highly advanced sailing skills to reach and settle islands, including Fiji, Tonga, Samoa, Tahiti, New Zealand (Maori) and later, in about 1000 BCE, Easter Island and Hawaii. Each Polynesian island has its own mythology, but certain consistencies among the stories make it possible to speak of Polynesian mythology in general. It is an animistic system in which gods are what they represent. The mythology contains familiar sexual themes such as the separation of copulating Heaven and Earth, creative incest, penis size and trickster eroticism.

The separation theme is nearly universal in Polynesia. The Maori version relates that Papa (female – Earth) and Rangi (male – Sky) once indulged in constant creative intercourse. But they clung together so closely that their creations had no room to move. One of their children, Tu (Tumatauenga), the embodiment of war, wanted to separate the parents by killing them. Another offspring, the storm god Tawhiri, wanted to leave things as they were. A third child, Tane, the spirit in plants and birds, wanted to separate the parents, leaving a space between them for sunlight and further creation. After several of the offspring of the primordial parents tried to separate them and failed, Tane lay on his back and pushed Papa away from Rangi with his feet, bringing into view creation itself. A war among the gods followed, with Tawhiri attempting to undermine order as he continues to do with his storms to this day. But Tane, Tu and Tangaroa, representing the sea (Ta'aroa in Tahiti, where he is the supreme god), prevailed and established peace. Similar myths exist in the Micronesian and Melanesian islands of the Pacific.

It is notable that the children of Papa and Rangi in this highly patriarchal culture are all male. The effect of this fact according to Sarah Dening in *The Mythology of Sex* was a deep Polynesian belief that the 'creative power' Polynesians call *mana* and we call 'libido' is essentially male, associated with Rangi. So it is that in traditional Polynesian societies a girl belonged to her father or husband and was considered a vessel for the creative semen of the male. To ensure fertility it was necessary to perform rituals – often explicitly erotic – which would arouse the *mana* of the male gods.

According to another Polynesian myth, Tane required a female partner for the procreation of humans. When his mother refused his advances, he created a female, Hine-hau-one (in Hawaii), out of sand or clay. The couple produced a daughter, Hine-titami, with whom Tane also copulated. This act of incest so disgusted the young Hine that she escaped to the underworld and became Hine-nui-te-po, the goddess of death.

In Hawaii and New Zealand some say that the last son of Papa and Rangi was the trickster and culture hero Maui. Others tell different stories of his parentage. In one myth his mother, whose identity is unclear, conceived him when she looked up at the sun. Most myths agree that when the child was born prematurely, his mother wrapped him in a lock of her hair – her top knot (*tikitki*) – and threw him into the sea. His father rescued him, however, and Maui immediately helped the people by slowing the sun down to provide more work time. Maui also created islands by raising them from the depths of the ocean, and tricked the goddess of fire into giving him – and humans – the secret of her being.

Sex is central in the Maui cycle. In a bizarre expression of the archetype of the hero's descent into the underworld, it is by way of a sexual act that Maui tries to overcome death itself. His goal is to enter the vagina of Hine-nui-te-po, the goddess of death, to travel through her body, and then to exit from her mouth, thus, in effect, overpowering her and removing death from the world. Death is stronger, however, and Maui is cut in half. In this act Maui attempts and fails to overcome the dangerous sexual power of the female, a version here of the vagina dentata archetype.

Before leaving the world, however, Maui lived a life that was focused to some extent on his and his primary enemy's genitals. In one story, Te Tuna the Eeel – Te Tuna sometimes being a term meaning 'penis' – was living with the goddess (or human) Hina. Hina became dissatisfied with Te Tuna and escaped from him in search of more satisfying sex. Arriving at the land of the Male Principle, she announced that she was the 'shameless pubic patch in search of love' (an embodiment of the vulva). Frightened of Te Tuna's power, however, the men sent Hina away. Finding her way finally to the place where Maui and his clan lived, Hina made the urgency of her desire clear and Maui's mother urged her son to take Hina as his wife.

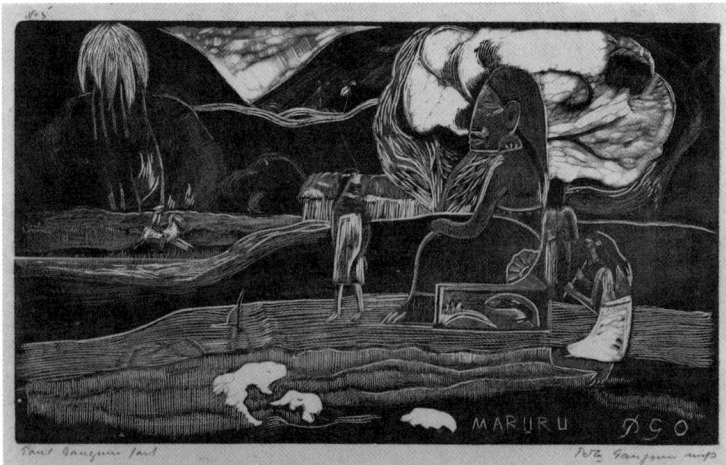

Paul Gauguin, *Maruru*, 1893–4, woodcut on paper, shows a Tahitian goddess.

Maui followed his mother's advice, and he and Hina experienced extreme passion. But some people told Te Tuna what was happening and eventually he approached Maui's land, his huge penis causing a tidal wave. Maui's mother urged her son to reveal his own member, which was said to be lopsided, to scare off Te Tuna and to stop the wave. This he did, and when Te Tuna arrived there was a great battle in which all of Te Tuna's companions were defeated. But Te Tuna was spared and he and Maui now agreed to share Hina as a wife. Things went well enough until the two 'husbands' decided to fight for sole ownership of their wife. While fighting, the two entered each other, perhaps reminding the reader of the sexual element in the struggle in Egyptian myth between Horus and Seth. Eventually Maui prevailed and cut off Te Tuna's head – that is, the source of his *mana*. Freud would call this castration. Maui buried – planted – the head, which eventually sprouted as the coconut plant, creating a staple of the Polynesian diet. The fascination with penis size is evident in the Maui myth as it is, for instance, in stories of African and Native American tricksters.

The Maui myth certainly has humorous aspects, as do all these trickster myths and such myths as those of Ares and Aphrodite or Zeus and his sexual conquests in Greece. It would be wrong, however, to dismiss this or any other Polynesian myth as mere entertainment. In this case, as the son of Rangi, the personification of the male principle, it is logical that Maui should use his penis, the genital symbol of that principle, in his struggle against rivals. The fact that ultimately Maui prevails as the sole husband of Hina indicates not only the establishment of a taboo against incest but a strong tradition of male dominance.

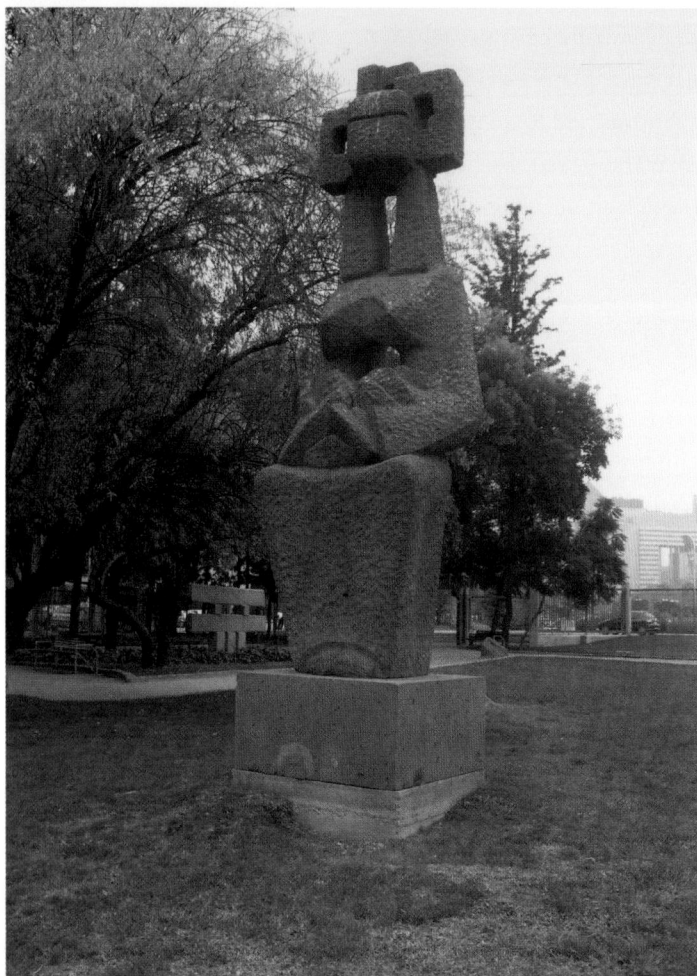

Marta Colvin, *Madre Tierra/Pachamama*, 1986, sculpture, Santiago, Chile.

Ten

The Americas

THERE IS NO definite knowledge as to how and when humans originally came to the Americas. The most common theory is that they arrived from Central Asia by way of the ice bridge to Alaska between 40,000 and 15,000 years ago, and that the Americas were the last land mass to be populated by Homo sapiens. Some people settled in the north, others made their way south into what is now Canada and the United States and on into Meso- and South America. There are several hundred cultural groups with their own languages and mythologies in the Americas. Many of these mythologies have significant sexual components.

Mesoamerican and South American Mythology

The mythologies of Mesoamerica and South America have been passed down orally and through pictographic/glyphic writing systems, some possibly among the oldest in the world, and through later works such as the Quiche Mayan *Popol Vuh* in the Spanish colonial period. Like all animistic traditions, South American and Mesoamerican mythologies in general recognize no separation between the spiritual and physical worlds, including when it comes to human sexuality.

As in other parts of the world, creation myths are common and in them sexual practices and attitudes regarding gender are established by supernatural events. Among the Yanomami of the Amazon forest, for example, there are myths about the creation of men and women which justify the position of males and females in Yanomami society. According to one myth it all began when Suhirina, a man in ancient times, shot an arrow at the moon. From the moon's blood as it flowed, men emerged and immediately fought violently with each other. After the fight, the men who were left longed for beings with which to relieve their sexual desires. One day a man found a ripe open fruit that had eyes. He threw it to the ground and it turned into a woman with a very large hairy vulva. The woman went with the men and had sex with each of them. The result was many daughters with whom the men had incestuous sex, producing the tribe now known as the Yanomami, who continue to believe in the importance of cross-cousin marrying. More importantly, this myth clearly establishes the male dominance and control of women which still prevails in Yanomami culture.

The Paraguayan Chamacoco people have a ceremony known as the Anaposo which reflects a myth also establishing a clear dominance of men over women. In this ceremony – a boy's initiation rite – spirits are revealed to be impersonated by men in masks. Women and pre-initiate boys are expected to consider the spirits to be real. It is believed that should women learn the truth about the impersonation, evil will be the result. In short, too much knowledge among women is considered destructive and dangerous. In a similar ritual among the Patagonian Selknam people, boys at initiation were told the secret of how to control women to prevent them from having the power they had in a previous age.

One myth associated with the Anaposo rite is an incest story in which a boy sees his mother's genitals, is overcome by desire, and seduces her. After the act, the mother demands to know the secret of the Anaposo and the boy reveals it to her. When the men find this out they kill all the women. One woman escapes. Without the women, the men are inflamed by unrequited desire. When the lone woman is discovered in a tree, the men try to climb up to her but are impeded by their erections, and they ejaculate on the tree. When the men finally catch the woman in another tree they rape her. Later she suggests that they dismember her and place her body parts around the sperm covered tree. These body parts the men take back home and eventually the body parts become new women.

Other creation myths also assume that the feminine aspect of nature gave birth to humanity. The Chorote of Bolivia, Argentina and Paraguay tell a story of the moon's wife Morning Star putting earth into her vagina and in that manner conceiving a son and a daughter, the first Chorotes. More often, the presence of women in the creation story is associated with their sexual power and the danger of that power. The ultimate expression of the dangerous female power is the vagina dentata archetype. The Toba people of Argentina say that men originated from the earth and that women came down from above bringing their destructive nature with them. They say that the women had two 'mouths' – one above and one between their legs. When one of the men approached one of the women to make her his wife, the woman bit off his genitals. The other men then threw stones at the women breaking their vaginal teeth.

The Yanomani say it was a woman who was the first human. She had a vagina with teeth with which she bit off any penis that entered there. As in most vagina dentata myths, a hero eventually defangs the vagina, establishing male control of that mysterious power.

The Chorote have an even more violent femme fatale myth. In this story, a man throws an axe at his wife, whom he suspects of evil intentions towards him. The axe grazes the woman and she licks the resulting blood with pleasure, confirming the man's suspicions that she has cannibal tendencies. When he is finally convinced by the woman to come down from the tree into her arms she breaks his neck and eats him, saving only his testicles which she cooks up in a dish for her friends.

A femme fatale story of the Yukuna people of the northern Amazon describes how a boy is rescued from a hole in a tree by a witch-like female figure with whom he has promised to have sex in return for the rescue. The boy rightly fears the witch and attempts to avoid intercourse with her. During the night, the witch begins to devour him by way of her anus. She almost succeeds, but when she gets as far as the boy's anus, the boy's anus devours *her*.

Male superiority is suggested in a Yanomami myth in which Omam, the creator, caught a female fish with whom he desired to have intercourse. To do so, however, he had to create her genitals. Even the vagina was created by a male. Similarly, some Mayans in Central America and the Yucatán of Mexico tell a story about the invention of female genitals. The story is part of a series of myths about the deer, an animal associated with both war and sex. It seems that the sun and moon had imprisoned the deer in a log in order to control him, but he escaped, and in a struggle that ensued he split the Moon Goddess, forming her vagina.

The Ona of Brazil say that the genitals of both men and women were made of peat by the culture hero Kenos. This is more in keeping with the creation myth of the Incas, in which the high god Viracocha or Pachacamac created the first man and woman out of clay. The woman was for some reason angry, so the creator had the first man make her pregnant. But as her first baby was born he cut it into many pieces and buried them. The planted body parts gave birth to the plants, which now feed the people.

There are myths in Mesoamerica and South America in which the female plays a more positive role, examples of the worldwide Great Mother archetype. One of the most popular of these goddesses is Pachamama, the fertility goddess worshipped by the Inca and other Andean cultures. Like other such goddesses, she is responsible for childbirth, the protection of women and the preservation of life. Others are Coatlicue and Cihuacoatl in Mexico, both of whom, like so many Great Goddesses elsewhere, have connections to serpent lore.

In Mesoamerica, one of the primary functions of sex in mythology is the conception of important deities or heroes, especially Huitzilopochtli and Quetzalcoatl. The goddess Coatlicue ('She of the Serpent-woven skirt'), the incarnation of the life force which animates everything in creation, lived on Serpent Mountain. Napping on the mountain one day, Coatlicue was impregnated miraculously by a ball of feathers (some say by the sun). Her already existing children were horrified by her pregnancy and would have killed her had she not suddenly delivered the fully armed Huitzilopochtli, the embodiment of war and the sun and the patron of the Aztecs. Huitzilopochtli defended his mother, killing many of his siblings in the process. This joining of the life force with military power was central to the Aztec identity.

The most popular of the Mesoamerican gods was Quetzalcoatl, the Feathered Serpent, the embodiment of the wind, of learning and of many other valuable attributes. There are numerous versions of his conception myth. The most common one says he was conceived when his virgin mother Chimilman swallowed an emerald.

As a serpent figure, Quetzalcoatl was also a symbol of fertility with phallic aspects. One myth has it that Coatlicue created humans from blood taken from Quetzalcoatl's penis in an act of creative sacrifice. The Mayan version of Quetzalcoatl, Kukulkan or Gukumatz, as the Feathered Serpent, acts with the god Tepeu in a creation myth to think the world into existence. In the process, the two gods use their power to separate Sky and Earth.

In another myth of the separation of the coupling Heaven and Earth, the Mosetene of Bolivia tell how a deity uses a giant snake to keep the couple apart. The snake is also at the centre of another fertility myth in Mesoamerica – a myth of the Zinecantecan culture of Chiapas in Mexico and of the Aztecs. There an important goddess was Cihuacoatl, or Quilaztli, a goddess of agriculture and of the creation of humans. It was Quetzalcoatl who brought bones from the land of the dead to Cihuacoatl. In this myth, it is Cihuacoatl rather than Coatlicue who grinds up the bones and fertilizes them with blood from Quetzalcoatl's penis. Cihuacoatl is often depicted with a phallic snake emerging from between her legs. As the purveyor of bad news about death, she is much like Kali in India. She represents the process in which death is a necessary part of existence.

Cihuacoatl has trickster aspects. She takes many forms and is highly sexual. In the Puebla area of Mexico she is called Matlacihualt or Mujer Enredadora ('Woman who Entraps'). In this impersonation she is sexually amoral, and she specializes in luring homosexual men into sex with her. Her vagina is at the back of her neck. It opens like a mouth, suggesting the vagina dentata motif, and if a man has sex with her he will become pregnant and give birth to a child that looks like excrement.

Tricksters play a familiar role in Mesoamerican and South American mythology and, as in many cultures, they double as

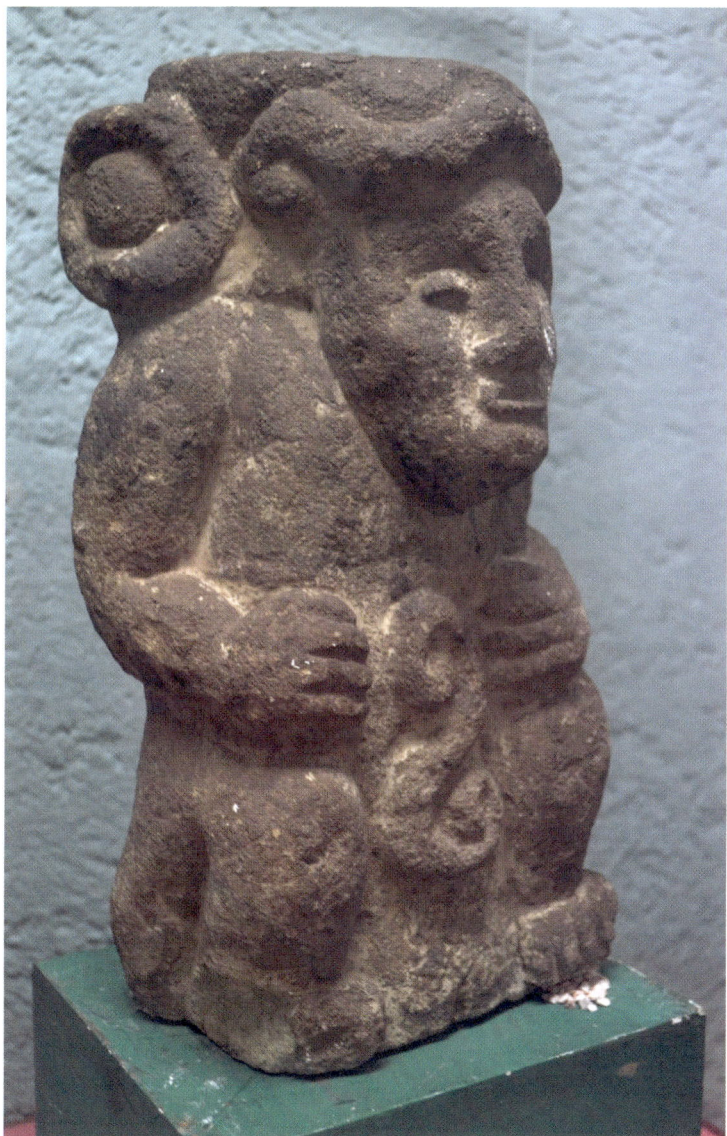

Stone sculpture of Cihuacoatl, 11th century.

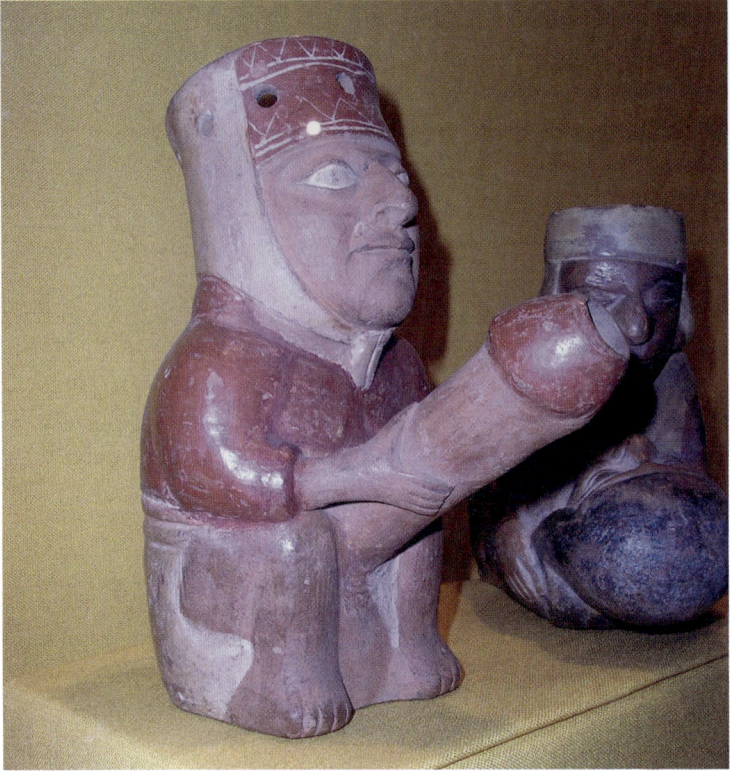

Kurupi, a Guarani trickster figure, pre-Columbian statuette.

culture heroes who teach the first people how to live. The Huichol of central Mexico, for instance, celebrate Kaurumari, who taught the people how to have intercourse. The primary characteristic of tricksters here as elsewhere is an unbridled sexual appetite.

The Tenetehara of Brazil, for example, tell many stories of the trickster Opossum. In one myth Opossum invites a pregnant woman into his hut and makes a hole in the roof over her bed mat so that rain falls on her, causing her to agree to share his bed, where he impregnates her with a second child. The result turns out to be a boon for the people. The child of Kaurumari will be a twin of the child already carried by the woman; these twins will be great heroes in the Tenetehara mythology.

Tricksters frequently become the butt of jokes. Kuwai is a trickster of the Columbian Amazonian people, the Cubeo. It was he who, as a cultural hero, taught the people how to experience sex. But having had to share one wife with his two brothers, he killed both the wife and the brothers and carved a new woman for himself out of wood. But this woman found his lovemaking unsatisfactory and took up with an anaconda, interestingly appropriate because the snake was the traditional companion for ancient goddesses.

In general, however, Mesoamerican and South American mythologies employ sex to establish the dominance of males over females, the assumption, especially in the case of South American mythology, being that female power – the mysterious power of sexual attraction – must be controlled. This conclusion is given

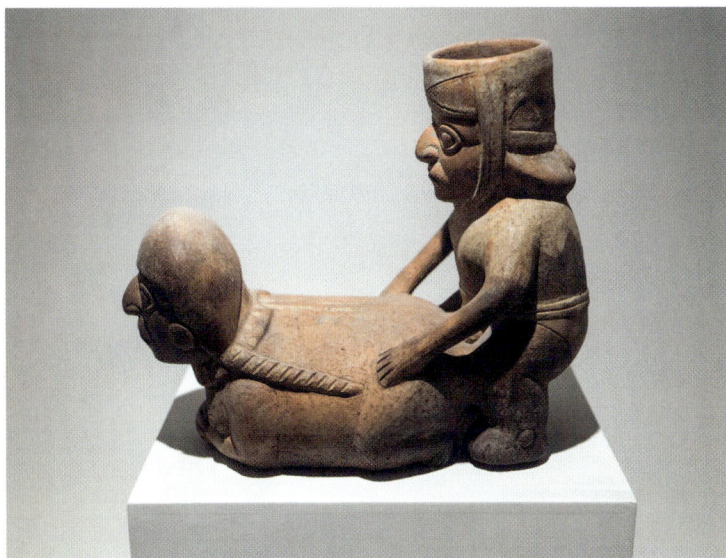

Moche erotic pottery, *c.* 1st century CE.

193

visual expression by the Moche of northern Peru, who are famous for their ceramic work and particularly for their erotic depictions. It is likely that these ceramics refer not only to sexual practices but to mythological stories. The figures are almost always depicted performing heterosexual acts, but anal penetration is more common than vaginal penetration. Fellatio sometimes occurs, but cunnilingus does not. Again, the tone here suggests male dominance of the female.

These little sculptures stand as representatives of the fact that in the mythology of the Southern part of the Americas, sex is revealed from a male perspective. They are clearly meant to entertain and are comic in the way ribald jokes among men are comic.

North American Mythology

North American mythologies represent many tribes who have in common an animistic approach to nature and to life in general. Several sexual themes present in mythologies elsewhere are here as well. These include the separation of a formerly united Earth Mother and Sky Father, miraculous conceptions, the presence of tricksters, and sexually based creation myths.

The theme of the separation of Heaven and Earth as expressed by Native Americans takes several highly original forms. The Zuni people of New Mexico place their myth in the 'womb' of the world where Earth Mother and Sky Father lay together so long that Earth Mother became so heavy with progeny that she had to push Sky Father away. Then her heaviness caused her to sink into the primeval waters below. But fearing for the safety of her unborn children, as mothers often do, she kept them inside of her. When she noticed a great bowl of water forming nearby she spat into the water, causing foam to form. She blew warm breath over the foam and some of the foam rose towards Sky Father, whose cold breathing on it caused rain that would bring sustenance to the children of Earth. As for the children, they could remain nestled in Earth's lap. In this way Earth and Sky cared for their progeny as separate but loving parents.

The Snohomish of the Northwest say the people were constantly banging their heads against the sky making things so uncomfortable that the tribes all got together and planted trees to keep the original couple apart.

North American separation myths are generally less violent than the separation myths of other cultures, such as the Polynesian, Egyptian and Greek. Many Indian tribes see the separation in terms of a maiden representing Earth falling away from a father representing Heaven or Sky. The Iroquoian-speaking peoples of eastern North America tell many versions of this myth. Typically, the maiden, living in a perfect world in the sky, becomes pregnant in a mysterious way and either falls or is pushed through a hole in Heaven. She floats down to maternal waters below and lands, usually on a turtle's back. Other animals dive into the waters to find soil, and out of that soil the maiden – now, in effect, Mother Earth – or her daughters create our world, a world characterized by fertility but also by the experience of death.

The point of this myth would seem to be that for creation to exist there must be a separation of Heaven and Earth. Heaven is static and deathless; Earth, to exist at all, must be creative and must be dominated by life cycles that include death. The Mother devours old life so that she can give birth to new life. In this sense, the Iroquoian Earth Mother resembles the Indian Great Goddess Devi in her forms as Durga or Kali. The sexuality that exists here is anything but prurient in nature. It is the sexuality that creates life and eventually death, and it is female oriented, a logical orientation for a culture which is matrilineal.

Often maidens in Native American myth are representatives of Mother Earth in that through their miraculous pregnancies and birthing they provide their people with some important boon. There are virgin birth stories in all corners of the continent. A particularly poignant one is told by the Tewa Indians who live near the Hopi Indians in Arizona. They tell how there was a beautiful girl who refused to marry. Her mother was a potter who spent most of her days making water jars out of clay. The girl often helped her mother by stomping on the wet clay to soften it. One day some of the clay entered her vagina and she became pregnant. The girl's mother was furious, not believing in her daughter's innocence. The girl's father, however, did not seem to mind. The girl gave birth, and her child was a living water jar with no arms or legs, just a mouth and eyes. After about twenty days the Water Jar Boy was big enough to ask his grandfather if he could go hunting with him. The grandfather pointed out that he was a water jar and would not be able to hunt. But the boy insisted and rolled along beside his grandfather. Suddenly he saw a rabbit and rolled down the hill after it. On the way, he hit a rock and broke apart. But out of the broken pieces of the jar a handsome young boy appeared, symbolizing his puberty. This boy went on to become a hero for the people. He searched for his father, the source of his identity, and discovered that his father was the Red Water Snake, an appropriate companion to the goddess representative who was his miraculously fertilized mother. With his father's help the boy prepared a place for the people to go to join their ancestors when they died. As in the Iroquoian myth, fertility and creativity are linked clearly to the cycles of life which include birth, puberty, a quest and death.

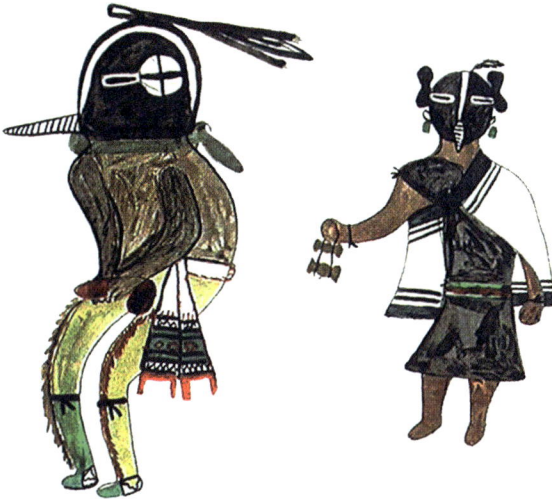

Ithyphallic Kokopelli Kachina with Mana, *c.* 540 CE, painting on animal skin.

As in most animistic cultures, most explicit sexuality is usually confined to stories of the trickster, of which North America has several, including the pre-Pueblan and Hopi figure Kokopelli, Iktomi the Spider on the Plains, Raven in the Northwest and Coyote everywhere.

Kokopelli was a fertility figure, responsible for agriculture and childbirth. He was hunchbacked, he played the flute, and typically he was depicted with an erection. It was said by the Hopi that he seduced young girls in their villages and that he carried unborn babies in his sack – babies that he might give to terrified girls. Like tricksters everywhere, he is all libido, all id.

Nowhere is this trickster libido more evident than in the tale of Iktome and the innocent maiden. Iktome had set his eyes on a beautiful and innocent young woman, so he changed his appearance into that of an old woman (tricksters are shape-shifters) and approached the young woman as she was about to cross a stream. 'Let's cross together,' said the trickster in an old woman's voice. When the two raised their dresses to cross, the girl commented on her companion's hairy legs: 'That happens with age,' Iktome said. As they raised their dresses higher with ever deepening water, the girl nervously noted the old lady's hairy backside. As the water grew still deeper and the dresses were raised still further, the girl noticed with some concern 'that thing hanging between your legs'. Iktome stopped and said, 'That's a growth put there by a sorcerer. It's heavy and it hurts and I wish I could be rid of it.' The girl suggested cutting it off, but Iktome cringed at the thought of that. 'I can only get rid of it by resting it between your legs,' he said. Wanting to be helpful, the innocent girl agreed to let her companion do as she had suggested. They finished crossing the stream and lay down on the soft grass where, soon enough, Iktome lay on top of the girl and entered her. 'Owe! that hurts,' cried the girl. 'It hurts me even more,' panted Iktome and in a while he rolled off. 'Look,' cried the girl. 'It worked; it's grown smaller.' A little later Iktome and the girl noticed that the thing had grown again so they repeated their 'curing' routine and repeated it several times after that. By the end of the day the girl was quite happy to be so helpful.

Penis fixation is common in the stories about the trickster Coyote. It was said that Coyote's penis was so long he kept it coiled up in a box. One tale has it that Coyote stood on a river bank, floated his penis slightly under water, and copulated with a young woman on the other side of the river.

The Paiutes tell one of many vagina dentata myths found in Native America. In this case a beautiful young woman approached the notorious Coyote and suggested that they have sex. The only trouble was that women's vaginas had teeth in those days. As Coyote knew that, he performed with great care. When the woman asked to make love again, Coyote carefully placed a rock in her vagina, which broke the teeth, and he used a rose bush to pull out the broken pieces. The woman shouted in pain, but now vaginas are the way men like them to be.

These stories are more like those of the trickster Maui than like those of the great god Shiva, whose phallus and sexuality generated worship rather than laughter. Native American trickster stories are decidedly male fantasies intended, like 'dirty jokes' everywhere, to entertain. The male fantasies involve sex, and centre on such issues as penis size and seduction. In many ways, these fantasies stand in contrast to Native American creation stories, which tend to celebrate the creative power of women and the earth.

An example of the archetype of the Great Goddess who is the source of creation is the Hopi figure, Spider Woman. In the beginning, there were only Tawa and the Sun God above and Spider Woman, the goddess of Earth below. In her form as Herewith, the Woman of Hard Substances, she became the lover of Tawa and gave birth to the sacred twins and to many other beings. It was she who wove life into existence. In her web, she gave life to Tawa's thoughts and the first humans were born – one a man like Tawa, one a woman like Huzruiwuhti. This first couple made love and produced the people who lived in Spider Woman's Earth until it was time for them to be born into the world through the little hole known as the *sipapu*, a hole found to this day in Hopi and other Pueblo kivas.

Other important Native American goddesses include Changing Woman of the largest Native American tribe, the Navajo of Arizona and New Mexico; White Painted Woman of the neighbouring and related Apache; White Buffalo Woman of the Sioux on the American plains; and Sedna among the Alaskan and Canadian Inuit (Eskimo). There are sexual components to each of these goddess stories. It is said that when Changing Woman had her first menses First Man and First Woman saw the event as one to be celebrated. They dressed the girl in a magnificent white dress, massaged her body and combed her hair. To this day Navajo and Apache girls repeat this process in a four-day ceremony (the *kinaalda*) at the onset of puberty. Navajo girls take on the healing powers of Changing Woman and Apache girls take on the powers of White Painted Woman during the event. This celebration of female sexuality stands in contrast to the usual emphasis in animistic and other cultures on the initiation of boys.

White Buffalo Woman is a major figure among the Sioux. When she first came to the people long ago a man desired her and tried to touch her sexually. Lightning struck and immediately turned him to ash. This was White Buffalo Woman's first lesson: she (and other women) must not be treated with disrespect. The goddess was, in effect, a culture hero. When she came to the people she opened her 'womb bag', gave them corn, taught them how to make fire for cooking, showed them how to pray and how to use the holy pipe. Smoke from the pipe was a bridge between the sacred earth below and the living breath of the Great Mystery above. The pipe ceremony today is considered a means of binding men and women together in a circle of love. When men and women marry they together hold the pipe and a cloth is wrapped around their hands, tying them together for life.

The Inuit Sedna is a different kind of figure. Her story is one of male–female relations gone bad, a familiar story of a 'good girl' being seduced by a 'bad boy'. Sedna was a beautiful young woman, much desired by the young men of her community. She lived happily with her father and avoided all temptations until one day a great and handsome sea bird convinced her to follow him to his home. Once at the bird's home Sedna saw how she had been duped. The bird was, in fact, an unclean fulmar chief who lived in a foul nest and treated her badly. In despair Sedna got a message to her father begging him to rescue her. The father did so after the winter ice melted, and he killed the fulmar. On the way home, the boat of Sedna and her father was threatened by a huge storm sent by the fulmar chief's followers. To avoid sinking, the father threw Sedna overboard. When the girl tried to hold on to the side of the boat the father cut off her fingers. At this point, the mistreated woman became a creator. Her chopped-off fingers turned into whales and other forms of sea life, and when she finally succeeded in returning to the boat she ordered her dogs to bite off her sleeping father's feet and hands. Then, after creating deer for the people, she left for a place under the world, where she rules today. Her father is there too – angry without feet and hands. When bad people die they go to Sedna's land and are forced to sleep with the father, who pinches them mercilessly.

An example of a creation story that celebrates the importance of men and women to each other in a sexual context is that of the Navajo. As in many southwestern creation myths, the Navajo describe how the people emerged in stages from one 'world' to another in Mother Earth until finally they arrived in the Fourth World. Here divine breath as wind blew on two ears of corn placed under buckskins and the corn became First Man and First Woman. The first couple had several sets of twins who learned to hunt and make useful things like pots and baskets. But First Woman wanted to establish a firm bond between men and women so she created the pleasure centres, the penis, the clitoris and the vagina. Coyote then came along and provided whiskers to make these parts more attractive and it became usual to keep them covered. One day First Man brought deer meat home for dinner and First Woman thanked her vagina. This irritated First Man who, after all, had done the hunting.

First Woman went on to explain that it was the vagina that inspired men to work – that without the enticement of the vagina they would do nothing. After a big argument in which First Woman said women had no real need of men, First Man stomped out and took all the men with him to live across the river from the women.

Things went well enough for a while. The men hunted and survived, but the women suffered from a lack of food. They sometimes came to the edge of the river and made lewd gestures to arouse the men's desires for them. The sexual longing of the men for the women and the women for the men grew as time went on. The women used all sorts of objects to satisfy themselves – everything from stones to cacti. The men sought relief in mud or deer livers. Finally, after four years, the wise owl pointed out to the men that they needed women to reproduce and that the women were beginning to starve and die. So, First Man sent a messenger to invite First Woman to the river bank, and when she came he apologized to her and the men and women happily rejoined each other. Later the men and women emerged together into this world.

Like many Indian tribes, the Navajo in their actual life approach sex modestly, but the fact that they can treat the sexuality of their sacred ancestors explicitly with an element of humour and without taking gender sides indicates an essential belief that sex is natural and beneficial and should be pleasurable to both men and women. The Navajo creation myth also reflects the matrilocal and matrilineal nature of Navajo culture. Lineage passes through the female line and a man when he marries moves to the land of his wife's family.

There is also a place in Native American culture for gender fluidity. A gender-neutral tradition in several Native American tribes is that of the 'Two Spirit' people. These are people who combine the identity of the two sexes. Thought of as neither men nor women they are often greatly respected as people who can perform multiple social roles. One myth in support of the Two Spirit idea is a Sioux story that it is the Great Spirit, the creator, who allocates gender roles. As a child is born, the creator points to baskets connoting femaleness and bows and arrows suggesting maleness. Occasionally, as the child of one gender reaches with a hand for the basket or the weapons, the creator switches the hand and the child chooses in such a way as to combine the two genders. The best known of the Two Spirit figures is the Zuni Lhamana, a much respected third gender person who typically wears both women's and men's clothing, who practises both male and female tasks and is depended on by the tribe as a mediator.

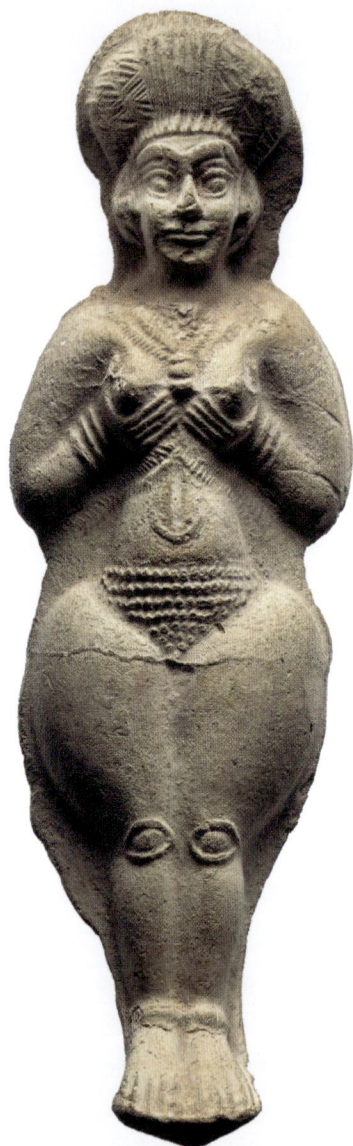

Probably an Elamite figure, 2nd or 3rd millennium BCE.

Conclusion:
Sex, Myth and the World

OUR NIGHT-TIME dreams reflect our personal lives and, at another level, more common human concerns. In the same way, the cultural dreams we call myths expose specific characteristics of the cultures that dream them as well as a more universal or archetypal human experience. In short, what means something for one culture can mean something quite different for another, but when a *world* mythology is considered comparatively, common elements suggest something – albeit something less specific – about humanity in general.

Several common elements stand out in this survey of sex in mythologies around the world. These include, for example, the separation of copulating Heaven and Earth early in the creation process, the sexual role of the Great Goddess, the miraculous conception, taboo sex (including bestiality, rape, homosexuality and incest), the femme fatale, genital – especially penis – fixation, and the lascivious trickster.

As plot makers, we humans need to know not only where we are going but where we came from. Most of us know who our parents are, but typically we want to know where we came from as a culture or a species. For this knowledge, we have tradition-ally turned to myths, and, given what we know of our own sexual creation, it makes sense according to mytho-logic that culturally we came from the sexual union of original cultural parents. In short, the original union of Mother Earth and Father Sky – Heaven and Earth – makes mythological sense since that union is based on the human understanding of the procreative process involving a man and a woman. The question then becomes why it is so urgent – as it is in so many mythologies – that Heaven and Earth be separated, putting an end to their creative sex act. In Mesopotamia, An and Ki are separated; in Egypt it is Geb and Nut; in Greece Gaia and Ouranos; in Polynesia Papa and Rangi; and in Canaan, El divides the original parents. In these cases, the separation is forced and even violent. Other separations are decidedly different. The prophets deny any union of Yahweh and Asherah in Israel. In China, the creator separates Heaven and Earth into Yin and Yang. In Africa, the division usually occurs when Heaven – personified by the creator – separates himself from Earth, becoming the *deus absconditus*, because of his disgust with humans. In North America, the separation is often associated with pregnancy. Once pregnant, the woman carries transitory life within herself; that is, with Earthly life comes death, and there is no place for death in Heaven.

The cultural implications in these myths can be surmised in various ways. In the Egyptian myth, for instance, we note the unusual fact that the Sky (Heaven) is female and the Earth male. Some have attributed this to the theory that the preferred sexual position for intercourse in Egypt was with the woman on top. The positions of Geb and Nut can also be traced to the importance of Egyptian goddesses and to the role of Nut (Sky) as a birthing female in the process of resurrection – that is, new birth – which was so central to Egyptian theology. The sub-Saharan myths of the *deus absconditus* suggest a sense that pervades African myth – a sense that life is difficult and that the people have been left to themselves to cope. The Hebrew prophets separated Yahweh from his popular association with Asherah to preserve the concept of monotheism. For the Chinese, Pangu's separating of the yolk and white of the original cosmic egg results in the Yin/Yang concept that was basic to a Chinese understanding of the world.

What most of these myths have in common is the sense that the separation of the original parents is necessary so that further creation can take place. The constant sexual union of the first parents is suffocating and ultimately selfish. The division of Father Sky and Mother Earth makes sense because only in their separated states can they concentrate on us and on our needs. Children tend not to want to see their parents in sexual congress because in that state parents concentrate on each other rather than on the children. When separate, Father Sky can send down rain, warmth and, in some cultures, spiritual guidance and even provide immortality. Mother Earth can nurture her children, even take them back into herself in the death that is so necessary for continued life. Another way of expressing this reality in contemporary terms might be to say that parents can be repressive in their caregiving or they can leave room for the self-development and creativity of their offspring.

Beginning at least as early as the Neolithic period, the sexual role of Mother Earth, the Great Goddess, has been a consistent mythological theme. The Goddess in her various forms has been essentially eponymous, that is associated with particular lands and cultures. In many mythologies, her sexual union with a male brings fertility and/or legitimacy to that culture. One can assume that the mysterious goddess of Çatal Hüyük represented her culture itself and was sexually related to the bull who seems always to be associated with her. Inanna of Sumer *was* the land, Sumer, waiting to be fertilized by lovemaking with Dumuzi. In India Devi takes many forms, but whether Kali or Parvati or Sarasvati or any number of other figures in union with divine figures such as Shiva and Vishnu, she is the Shakti, the divine cosmic energy without which the power of divinity cannot take form. When in Irish mythology Morrigan sleeps with the Dagda or the Irish Kings mate with the eponymous Irish queens or *Matres*, sovereignty and the reality of Ireland itself is established. The same is true in Wales when Pwyll marries the goddess Rhiannon, or in Polynesia when Kunapipi mates symbolically with her companion snake and creates the land. In Native North America, the goddess maiden who falls from the sky carries the results of her union with divinity within her and can establish creation on Earth, which is to say, on herself. Each of these and many other examples of union with the Earth Mother is related to the establishment of given cultures. But the central universal meaning is also clear. The Great Goddess is the Earth Goddess, and the fertility and nurturing power of earth are essential to life. Nevertheless, the male-dominated patriarchal world has taken great pains to obliterate the Great Goddess. In her Mesopotamian form as Tiamat she was killed and dismembered by the Babylonian city god Marduk; in Greece she was turned into the vamp Aphrodite or the masculinized Athene and Artemis and replaced as the guardian of Delphi by the god Apollo; in the Hebrew Bible she was displaced entirely by a wifeless god.

Yet somehow the Goddess has survived. Devi – often in sexual roles as Parvati in Shiva's embrace or as Kali dancing over his prostate body – remains a powerful figure in India's religious life today. In Christianity the cult of the Goddess, albeit as a virgin, is present as a de facto reality in Catholic churches everywhere. The continued existence of the virgin birth myth, despite a reasonable scepticism regarding it, is a way in which the demand of the Goddess for her rightful place is expressed. 'Ultimately,' she says, 'birth and life come from me; my body is the portal, the way.' In short, although the cult of virginity is tied to the male's understanding that the female is his possession – his alone – the virgin birth myth expresses a hope of independence and even feminist warning to the male that he is not as important as he thinks he is. This warning is repeated in the Gaia theory of modern science, a theory that takes its name from the Greek creator goddess and postulates that Earth will survive in one form or another however we who live on her destroy ourselves by our environmentally disastrous actions.

The Goddess and a human need to release sex from the idea of sin persists in animistic cultures. In southwestern Native America, for instance, the tiny *sipapu* holes in the floors of the kiva symbolize the place of entry of the people into this world from the goddess mother, an emergence told about in several tribal creation myths. These myths are made real and immediate by the Kachina (spirit figures) who emerge in ceremonies from a second symbolic birthing hole at the top of the kiva into the living world of the pueblo plaza. The Kachina are dancing visitors from the animating spirit world of the Goddess.

The motif of the miraculous conception is in some ways an extension of the goddess story. The miraculous conception is generally reserved for heroes, culture heroes, and for gods who act in those roles. Isis conceives Horus as she flutters as a bird over the dead body of the murdered Osiris. The cultural meaning here is clearly related to the Egyptian fixation on life after death. Isaac and John the Baptist are born of barren mothers, symbolizing the power of the Abrahamic God. Jesus is born of the union between a virgin and a mysterious being said to be the Holy Spirit. Chinese culture heroes are almost always miraculously conceived. Qi's mother conceived when she stepped in a footprint left by the supreme deity; the Polynesian trickster Maui was conceived when his mother looked at the sun; the Buddha's mother, Maya, conceived her son through contact with a white elephant in a dream; the Irish hero Cúchulainn was miraculously conceived through the agency of the god Lugh as a fly in Dechtire's drink; the Indian man god Krishna was conceived when the great god Vishnu entered the womb of Devaki; in Mesoamerica, the god Huitzilopochtli was conceived by Coatlicue and a ball of feathers or the sun, and Chimilman swallowed an emerald to be impregnated with Quetzalcoatl. Native North Americans tell many miraculous conception stories, including the one of the maiden who is 'entered' by a bit of clay, causing her to give birth to a water jar. These tales reflect cultural concerns. Cúchulainn and Krishna are avatars of divine beings. The sun is central to Polynesian and Mesoamerican life. For the Tewa Native Americans, known for their pottery, a piece of clay is animated by spirit and thus contains the potential for life.

The miraculous conception also reflects a tendency to evade the connection between sex and the birth of heroes. It expresses a universal longing for the presence of divinity in the world. Although divinity can only have human dimensions if it enters the world by way of human female genitals, the implantation of the sacred seed does not involve ordinary sex. By divorcing the conception of the hero from the ordinary sexual activity of two human parents, the myth-makers emphasize that the hero, the representative of a new beginning, belongs to everyone. But by doing so they also perpetuate the idea that ordinary sex acts are somehow unclean or shameful, an idea that has persisted in much of human society.

The negative sense of human sexuality is made especially apparent in myths of taboo sex – stories of bestiality, rape, incest and other

forbidden activities. Examples of bestiality include those of the Minoan
queen Pasiphae and the Great Bull, Zeus as a bull abducting Europa,
Zeus as a swan having his way with Leda, and Loki becoming female
and being mounted and made pregnant by a stallion. Scholars have
suggested that these myths suggest bestiality practices in ancient
cultures, especially relating to fertility and totem rituals.

Rape is more common, often in conjunction with incest. Gilgamesh asserts his *droit de seigneur* with the newly married women of
Uruk; Zeus rapes Leda, Europa and many others; Hades abducts and
rapes his niece Persephone; Poseidon rapes his sister Demeter and
Medusa as well; the Dogon creator Amma rapes his creation, Earth.
These rapes have various cultural implications. In the case of the
rapes carried out by the Olympian gods, the myth-makers reflect the
realities of a highly patriarchal society. Ordinary people – particularly women – were at the mercy of those above them; the gods
could do what they pleased with humans.

Homosexuality, either actual or implied, is present in several
mythologies. Scholars argue as to whether various close relationships
in myths between men should be considered homosexual in nature.
Gilgamesh and Enkidu, Achilles and Patroclus, David and Jonathan
are examples. It could be argued that these relationships simply represent a tendency in Greek and other cultures to elevate the nature of
male friendship over male–female relations. Homosexual relationships, such as the violent one between Seth and Horus in Egypt, and
the abduction of the boy, Ganymedes, by Zeus, and even the more
romantic ones between the young Hyacinth and Apollo and Herakles
and the youthful Hylas, also reflect a general view of many cultures,
including those of ancient China, Japan, Greece and Egypt and some
today, that sex in certain circumstances between a man and a boy is
acceptable, and that though penetration of another male is manly

enough, the reception of penetration beyond the age of adolescence is effeminate and deplorable.

Lesbian and transgender sex do not play major roles in mythology. There are rare examples, as in the case of Zeus turning himself into the goddess Artemis so that he can have sex in a lesbian context with the beautiful follower of Artemis, Callisto. Another transgender myth is that of Tiresias, who experienced sex as both a man and a woman. In both cases the changes that occur are based not on a desire to change genders but rather on circumstantial convenience or divine disapproval. The same is true of the more comic transgender experiences of Herakles and Achilles in Greek mythology, and Loki and Thor in Norse mythology. In the case of the Androgyne – Hermaphroditus in Greece, for instance, and sometimes even great gods such as the Shiva as Parvati combined as Ardhanarisvara – what seems perverse becomes a symbol of a state of wholeness longed for in sexual union.

The most common form of taboo sex in mythologies is incest. Incest is a natural extension of the condition of the world at the beginning of creation. If there are only brothers and sisters in existence incest will be inevitable, as in the cases, for instance, of the Dogon Nummo twins, Fuxi and Nuwa in China, Izanami and Izanagi in Japan, the Djanggawuls in Australia and the original Yanonami in South America. In other cases, the mythical incest is associated with cultural incest not considered a taboo. The Egyptian relationships between Geb and Nut or Osiris and Isis are in keeping with the approved pharaonic marriages between brother and sister. In still other cases the incest is the result of attitudes of gods who consider themselves to be outside of the requirements of any moral code. The Greek Olympians are a prime example. Not only do Olympians rape each other, they have consensual familial sex. Hermes and Aphrodite had a relationship that resulted in a child, Hermaphroditus. Aphrodite also had sex with Dionysos and more famously with her brother Ares. These two were caught in a net by the goddess's husband Hephaistos, much to the merriment but hardly the outrage of the rest of the Olympian family.

Mythical incest can be reprehensible but productive, an intricate part of creation itself. Prajapati, an Indian creator, and others in Vedic mythology, are condemned for their incestuous acts that took place before incest was even a concept. The same is true of Tane in Polynesia, who was refused by his mother but who copulated creatively with his daughter and was condemned by his wife, Hine. In Wales, the incestuous relationship of Gwydion and his sister Aranrhad resulted in the sea god Dylan.

Other acts of incest in mythology are clearly taboo acts standing as examples of evil. Lot and his daughters in the Bible and Myrrah in Greek mythology are women who trick their fathers into sex with them and are clearly negative examples, as is the biblical Amnon, who seduced his sister Tamar.

The most famous of incestuous acts is that of Oedipus, who literally did not know what he was doing but who was punished anyway. Once again, this is a myth that reflects the Greek sense of the arbitrariness of the gods and the inflexibility of divine prophecy and justice. Sex is always a part of our being, and whatever the circumstances, it will find a way of expressing itself, almost always with significant consequences. Perhaps the fascination with forbidden sex – a fascination that has always persisted in pornography as well as in mythologies – reflects the universal sense of the power of the sex drive and its ability to transcend even the strictest of social mores, laws and traditions.

An important composite figure in the world sex myth who also represents the pure power of sex – often of the forbidden type – is the femme fatale, the sexually dangerous woman. The list of these figures, beginning with the Mesopotamian Ishtar who tried to seduce Gilgamesh, is long, and the women are consistent in their effect. Essentially what they do is undermine the strength and the destiny of men through sexual attraction. Nowhere is this femme fatale archetype stronger than in the biblical tradition. Eve eats of the forbidden fruit in the Garden of Eden and convinces her husband to do the same. Before disobeying the order 'they were both naked, the man and his wife, and were not ashamed'. After the disobedience 'the eyes of them both were opened, and they knew that they *were* naked; and they sewed fig leaves together, and made themselves aprons.' Clearly the Bible sees Eve's sin as one leading to Adam's and then to sexual shame in general. In the Talmudic tradition, an even worse femme fatale associated with Adam is Lilith, who insisted on having intercourse while on top of Adam. Eve and Lilith are followed in the Bible by a host of women – Jezebel, Delilah, Bathsheba and Salome, for example – who weaken their men or lead them through sexual desire into sin. The biblical prophets saw the Canaanite Asherah as a sexual threat to their religion and culture. Among the Greeks Aphrodite was the prime femme fatale. Helen of Troy, Calypso, Circe and Medea also used sex to undermine manly missions. For Virgil, Dido played the role of a femme fatale in that her sexual attraction almost deterred Aeneas from the sacred purpose of his quest to found Rome, the new Troy. In Ireland Morrigan became the femme fatale when she tried to seduce Cúchulainn. Queen Medb is another Irish femme fatale; her selfish acts caused the great war of the *Tain Bo Cuailnge*. A popular Arthurian femme fatale is Morgan le Fay. Perhaps the most undisguised femmes fatales are the vagina dentata of Native America, Polynesia, India, Japan, South America and elsewhere, who attract men and then literally chew up their penises.

Few things are more frightening to men than the loss of the penis. The penis is the symbol of male power and sexual prowess in patriarchal societies. In many cultures, simply to have a penis is to have the potential for power and dominance. Not to have one in Freudian mythology, for example, is to have 'penis envy'. The fixation on the penis is a phenomenon that begins as far back as the Palaeolithic cave paintings and is a consistent presence in world mythology. In the Heliopolis system in Egypt the high god masturbated the world into existence. As in other patriarchal cultures, the penis is the logical expression of the creator's generative powers. The penis of El reaches out to create in Canaan, as does the phallus of the Vedic creator in India. The male organ is celebrated in phallic stone columns in many parts of the ancient world from Harappa to Ireland, Canaan to Polynesia. In Egypt, Isis was said to have made a model of the penis of her dead husband Osiris, and in Osiris celebrations the god's phallus was carried in ritual processions. In Greece, the phallus of Dionysos was processed during the Dionysiad festival in Athens, and the protective penis of Hermes stood erect on herms in front of doors and other liminal spaces. Penis length was celebrated in ubiquitous Greek and Roman ithyphallic depictions of Satyrs and of Dionysos' companion, Silenus. In Rome, flying phalli were featured in Mars festivals remembering the huge phallus that impregnated a slave girl and engendered Romulus and Remus. The ritual celebrations of the phallus in Egypt, Greece, Rome and Japan, and the myths that support these celebrations, were clearly reflective of a belief in patriarchal societies of male superiority symbolized by the generative organ.

In Hebrew mythology, the revered penis is central to a similar belief. The Book of Deuteronomy declares that a woman who damages a man's genitals should have her hand cut off. Castrated men

– even castrated animals – were forbidden entrance to temple rituals. Noah's son is condemned for seeing his father's genitals. The reverence of the penis is, of course, most evident in the rite of circumcision, a rite that existed in ancient Egypt and elsewhere in Africa as well, but which for the Hebrews became a necessary and central ritual. The circumcised penis in the Jewish tradition is the symbol of membership in a community established by God in his interaction with Abraham. The same symbol applies to Islam, another Abrahamic religion under the same god. For Christianity, as developed by Paul of Tarsus and others, physical circumcision was not considered necessary and, in fact, among Christians, where sex has been more adamantly associated with sin than in Judaism and Islam, the penis has played less of a defining or symbolic role except insofar as the necessity of hiding it is symbolic of that sense of its role in sin.

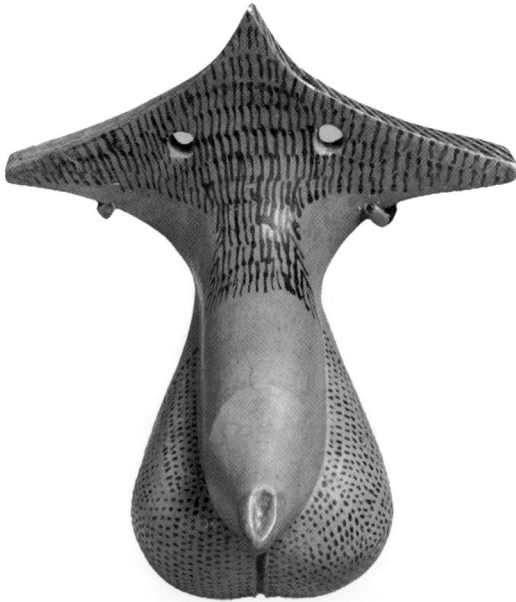

Greek terracotta vase in the shape of a phallus, 550–500 BCE.

In India, the phallus of Shiva, the lingam, is evident everywhere. It stands in conjunction with the yoni of the goddess and is represented in various states on temple walls. In one myth, its endless length becomes the symbol of the god's infinite power and significance. Penis length is a frequent theme in many cultures. In Australian myths such as those of the Djanggawul, the long Djanggawul (penis) plays an important role in the 'dreaming' creation. Among other peoples – those of sub-Saharan Africa, Polynesia and Native North America, for instance, penis length is treated comically, usually in association with trickster figures.

Tricksters are ubiquitous in the sexual mythology of the world. Whether Enki filling his wife, his children and his grandchildren – all symbolizing the marshes of Mesopotamia – with his semen, the Devil enticing Eve and Adam to eat the forbidden fruit, or Ananse and Maui and Coyote performing their extraordinary sexual feats, the trickster is there representing the amoral pre-conscious state of being. The trickster is a relief valve, the id/libido unfettered by the so-called moral and 'family' standards. He is the embodiment of the sexual urge that is necessary for the continuance of procreation and life itself. The trickster stands against the dominant patriarchal consciousness which tends to equate sex with sin and danger.

A question that inevitably follows a survey of sex in the world of myth is what role the elements revealed by that survey play in our world today. The ancient myths are most evidently thriving in the practice of extant religions related to them. The literal effect that the myths have on the practitioners of these religions depends on what might be called the level of belief. For a fundamentalist follower of the god Shiva in India, the story of the god's infinitely long phallus would have more literal meaning than it would for the Vedantic Hindu who would be likely to see the phallus as a metaphor. The same difference applies to the understanding of people of the Abrahamic faiths about the sexuality of Adam and Eve and particularly to Christians about the virginity of Mary. That myths associated with religions do have power and relevance in the world today becomes evident when we consider the fact that humans continue to turn to them in worship and even to fight wars over their interpretation.

As operative as sexual myths are in religious practice and belief, they also affect secular life. Taboo sex has always fascinated us, and literature and pornography are rife with examples of brother–sister, father–daughter and mother–son sex. A psychological version of the separation myth, for example, was created by Freud in his famous Oedipus complex, in which the child is jealous of his father and sexually attracted to his mother. As in the case of all myths, we react to this modern myth with varying degrees of literal belief. The same is true when we consider Freud's theories of penis envy or Jungian theories on the connection between the Great Goddess and human approaches to sex.

Perhaps more important is the effect myths have on the way human beings look at each other sexually, how the genders act together, for instance, or how homosexuality or transgenderism are treated. In all the mythologies discussed in this survey of sex in world mythology, several telling points of view stand out. However powerful the Great Mother Goddess, the myths tell us that the universe is ruled by beings representing a male perspective based on physical power. This power often stands in direct opposition to the sexual power associated with the female. Women in myth are often seen by men as a threat, simply because their sexual attraction is strong and thus capable of leading them astray. The femme fatale archetype is the mythological justification for male suppression of the female in what is seen essentially as self-defence: 'The Devil made me do it and the Devil is in the woman.'

It can be argued that the femme fatale myth has had more of an effect on human societies and on human society than any other myth. It is the femme fatale who has sealed the fate of women as the inferior gender. Blaming women from Eve and Pandora onwards for using sex to lead men away from their moral and reasonable selves, men have fought back. To undermine female sexual power men have restricted the movement and power of women by establishing a cult of virginity, by attaching women to individual men through marriage and property laws, by forcing women to cover themselves from view, by limiting their contact with other men, by genital mutilation and by a certain brutality in sexual relations. An examination of the highly popular pastime of pornography, for instance, will show that men take pleasure in humiliating women, in using the penis to 'bang', 'pound', 'punish', 'nail' and 'gag' them.

It should be noted, however, that the rise of feminism in religious traditions and elsewhere suggests the resistance of the feminine to arbitrary masculine power. For the patriarchal male, the body of a woman has been a metaphor for or symbol of sex, and from that point of view, the presence of women in religious, ritualistic roles usually filled by men is often seen as a confusion of sex and religion. Today in the Abrahamic traditions, especially reformed elements of Judaism and Christianity, that view is being challenged as misogynistic and outmoded. Feminism can, of course, lead to mythological concepts such as God 'Our Mother' rather than 'Our Father'. And such metaphors simply substitute one limiting view of deity for another. Gender fluidity is a more modern concept and one that will almost certainly require changes in sexual metaphors applied to the mythical world of religion.

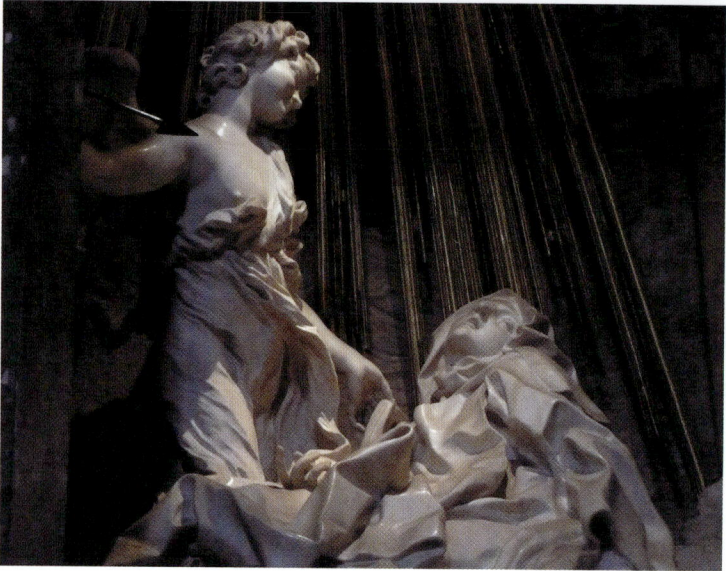

Gian Lorenzo Bernini, *The Ecstasy of Saint Teresa*, c. 1650,
white marble sculpture.

Whatever the future holds for the role of sex in our mythologies,
it helps to remember that the figures and situations conjured up in
our dreams are all aspects of ourselves. This fact applies to both
our personal and collective dreams. The separation of Heaven and
Earth, the role of the Great Goddess, the concept of the miraculous
conception, taboo sex, the femme fatale, genital – especially penis –
fixation and the lascivious trickster are all parts of our psychic lives
and they suggest a human failing, a tendency to equate sex with
danger and evil, and a loss of the kind of vision expressed in the
ancient hymns of Inanna, the 'Song of Songs', or the depictions of
the union of Shiva and Parvati.

Ultimately, sex in the world of myth comments on the great
power of sex, inner drives that can be expressed metaphorically
through the violent acts of Zeus, the destructive but uncontrollable

passions of Pasiphae or Tristan, the love of Cúchulainn for Fergia, the foolish and amoral escapades of Coyote, the exacting demands of Kali or the cruel devices of Morgan le Fay. These are all aspects of us, both males and females.

Finally, even when a mythology tends to avoid or suppress sexual tales and images, as Christianity has done, sex has a way of coming to the surface. Bernini's great painting of the ecstasy of St Teresa of Avila, for instance, captures the sexual dimension of Teresa's love of her God. The sixteenth-century Spanish mystic John of the Cross, in the tradition of the Sumerian hymns to Inanna, the 'Song of Songs', the poetry of the Muslim Sufi sage Jalaladin Rumi, and others, used erotic imagery to convey his mystical relationship with the same god:

> How gently and lovingly
> you wake in my heart,
> where in secret you dwell alone;
> and in your sweet breathing,
> filled with good and glory,
> how tenderly you swell my heart with love.

The seventeenth-century English metaphysical poet John Donne, a clergyman, also discovered that only sexual imagery, derived from the ecstatic experience of the human body, could express the divine ecstasy of his mythic world:

> Batter my heart, three-person'd God, for you
> As yet but knock, breathe, shine, and seek to mend;
> That I may rise and stand, o'erthrow me, and bend
> Your force to break, blow, burn, and make me new.

SEX IN THE WORLD OF MYTH

I, like an usurp'd town to another due,
Labour to admit you, but oh, to no end;
Reason, your viceroy in me, me should defend,
But is captiv'd, and proves weak or untrue.
Yet dearly I love you, and would be lov'd fain,
But am betroth'd unto your enemy;
Divorce me, untie or break that knot again,
Take me to you, imprison me, for I,
Except you enthrall me, never shall be free,
Nor ever chaste, except you ravish me.

Bernini, John of the Cross and Donne reiterate in their works what myth-makers have always known: that sex – however distorted – is the human experience that most clearly expresses the longings and fears that make us who we are.

ACKNOWLEDGEMENTS

I wish to thank Ben Hayes for his original encouragement and editing in connection with this book and all the staff at Reaktion Books for their support in its realization.

PHOTO ACKNOWLEDGEMENTS

The author and the publishers wish to express their thanks to the below sources of illustrative material and / or permission to reproduce it.

Alamy: pp. 42 (Art Collection 3), 46 (Paul Fearn), 80 (Art Collection), 161 (Paul Fearn), 163 (Tribune Content Agency LLC), 166 (Ariadne Van Zandbergen); Juan Cabré Aguiló: p. 12; Jenniferboyer: p. 131; British Library: p. 164; © The Trustees of the British Museum, London: pp. 33, 100, 116; Mariel Corona: p. 19; Chris73: p. 64; Jean-Pierre Dalbéra: p. 119; Deccan School: p. 110; G41rn8: p. 109; Getty Images: pp. 34 (CM Dixon/Print Collector), 118 (Dushyant Thakur Photography); Hispalois: p. 115; Institute for the Study of the Ancient World: p. 90; The Israel Museum: p. 24; Jamain: p. 86; The Metropolitan Museum of Art, New York: pp. 55, 182, 204, 216; Stealth3327: p. 162; Spud Murphy from Sydney, Australia: p. 125; NK: p. 13; Nessy-Pick: p. 126; Niels from Amsterdam: p. 173; Marie-Lan Nguyen: pp. 77, 81; Fernandopascullo: p. 192; Penarc: p. 184; Pinkpasty: p. 146; Rama: pp. 18, 44; © José Luiz Bernardes Ribeiro: p. 85; WolfgangRieger: p. 68; Roweromaniak: p. 15; Sandstein: p. 40; Thomas Schoch: pp. 176, 177, 178; Shutterstock: p. 193 (saiko3p); Sid Storm: p.14; Teufelbeutel: p. 129; Kim Traynor: p. 92; Walters Art Museum, Baltimore: pp. 36, 117; Welleschik: p. 220.

BIBLIOGRAPHY

Ackermann, Susan, *When Heroes Love: The Ambiguity of Eros in the Stories of Gilgamesh and David* (New York, 2006)

Akerly, Ben Edward, *The X-rated Bible: An Irreverent Survey of Sex in the Scriptures* (Port Townsend, WA, 1998)

Angulo, Javier, and Marcos Garcia Diez, *Sexo en piedra* (Sex in Stone) (Madrid, 2006)

Armstrong, Karen, *A History of God* (New York, 1991)

Aurobindo, Sri, *The Secret of the Veda* (New Delhi, 1998)

Berndt, Ronald Murray, *Kunapipi: A Study of an Australian Aboriginal Religious Cult* (Melbourne, 1951)

Bierhorst, John, *The Mythology of South America* (Oxford and New York, 1988)

Bisson, Luc, *Sexual Ambivalence: Androgyny and Hermaphroditism in Graeco-Roman Antiquity*, trans. Janet Lloyd (Berkeley, CA, 2002)

Bonnefoy, Yves, *Asian Mythologies*, trans. Wendy Doniger (Chicago, IL, 1993)

Brown, W. Norman, 'The Creation Myth of the Rig Veda', *Journal of the American Oriental Society*, 2 (June 1942)

Campbell, Joseph, *Goddesses: Mysteries of the Feminine Divine*, ed. Safron Rossi (Novato, CA, 2013)

——, *The Hero with a Thousand Faces* (Princeton, NJ, 1974)

——, *The Masks of God*, 4 vols (New York, 1968)

Cashford, Jules, *The Myth of the Goddess: Evolution of an Image* (New York, 1991)

Chrystal, Paul, *In Bed with the Ancient Greeks: Sex and Sexuality in Ancient Greece* (Amberley, Stroud, 2016)

Clark, R. T. Rundle, *Myth and Symbol in Ancient Egypt* (London, 1959)

Coogan, Michael David, ed. and trans., *Stories from Ancient Canaan*
(Louisville, KY, 1978)
Craig, Robert D., *Handbook of Polynesian Mythology* (Santa Barbara,
CA, 2004)
Cross, T. P., and C. H. Slover, *Ancient Irish Tales* (Lanham, MD, 1969)
Crossley-Holland, Kevin, *The Norse Myths* (New York, 1980)
Dalley, Stephanie, ed. and trans., *Myths from Mesopotamia: Creation,
The Flood, Gilgamesh, and Others* (New York and Oxford, 2008)
Dening, Sarah, *The Mythology of Sex* (New York, 1996)
Doniger, Wendy, *The Hindus: An Alternative History* (Oxford, 2010)
——, *Redeeming the Kamasutra* (Oxford, 2016)
——, *Textual Sources for the Study of Hinduism* (Manchester, 1988)
Doty, William G., *Mythography: The Study of Myths and Rituals*
(Tuscaloosa, AL, 2000)
Douglas, Mary, *Purity and Danger: An Analysis of the Concepts of Pollution
and Taboo* (London, 1984)
——, and Phyllis Kaberry, *Man in Africa* (New York, 1971)
Elledge, Jim, *Gay, Lesbian, Bisexual, and Transgender Myths: From the
Arapaho to the Zuni* (New York, 2002)
Erdoes, Richard, and Alfonso Ortiz, eds, *American Indian Myths and
Legends* (New York, 1984)
Fang Fu, Ruan, with Molleen Matsumura, *Sex in China: Studies in Sexuality
in Chinese Culture* (New York, 1991)
Fee, Christopher, and David A. Leeming, *Gods, Heroes, and Kings:
The Battle for Mythic Britain* (New York and Oxford, 2001)
Foucault, Michel, *The History of Sexuality*, 3 vols (New York, 1986)
Gates, Henry Louis, *The Signifying Monkey: A Theory of African-American
Literary Criticism* (Oxford and New York, 2014)
Gimbutas, Marija, *The Language of the Goddess* (London, 1989)
Girardot, N. J., *Myth and Meaning in Early Taoism: The Theme of Chaos
(hun-tun)* (Berkley, CA, 1983)
Graves, Robert, *The White Goddess* (New York, 1958)
Grene, David, and Richard Lattimore, ed. and trans., *Greek Tragedies*,
3 vols (Chicago, IL, 1992)
Griaule, Marcel, *Conversations with Ogotemmeli: An Introduction to Dogon
Religious Ideas* (Oxford, 1975)
Hansen, William, *Classical Mythology* (Oxford and New York, 2004)
Hart, Eloise, 'Inanna, Queen of Heaven and Earth', *Sunrise* (October/
November 2002)
Hesiod, *Theogony* and *Works and Days* (Oxford and New York, 1988)

Highwater, Jamake, *Myth and Sexuality* (New York, 1990)

Homer, *Iliad,* trans. Barry B. Powell (Oxford and New York, 2014)

——, *Odyssey,* trans. Robert Fitzgerald (New York, 1961)

Huainanzi, ed. and trans. John S. Major, Sarah A. Queen, Andrew Seth Meyer and Harold D. Roth (New York, 2010)

Hunt, Eva, *The Transformation of the Hummingbird: Cultural Roots of a Zinacantecan Mythical Poem* (Ithaca, NY, 1977)

Knipe, Rita, *The Water of Life: A Jungian Journey Through Hawaiian Myth* (Honolulu, HI, 1989)

Koch, John T., and John Carey, *The Celtic Heroic Age: Literary Sources for Ancient Celtic Europe and Early Ireland and Wales* (Aberystwyth, 2003)

Kramer, Samuel Noah, *Mythologies of the Ancient World* (Chicago, IL, 1961)

——, *Sumerian Mythology: A Study of Spiritual Achievement in the Third Millennium B.C.* (Philadelphia, PA, 1972)

——, and John Maier, *Myths of Enki: The Crafty God* (Oxford and New York, 1989)

Leeming, David A., *Creation Myths of the World*, 2 vols (Santa Barbara, CA, 2009)

——, *A Dictionary of Asian Mythology* (New York and Oxford, 2001)

——, *From Olympus to Camelot: The World of European Mythology* (New York and Oxford, 2003)

——, *Jealous Gods and Chosen People: The Mythology of the Middle East* (New York and Oxford, 2004)

——, *Medusa: In the Mirror of Time* (London, 2013)

——, *Myth: A Biography of Belief* (New York and Oxford, 2002)

——, *Mythology: The Voyage of the Hero* (New York and Oxford, 1998)

——, *The Oxford Companion to World Mythology* (New York and Oxford, 2005)

——, *The World of Myth* (New York and Oxford, 2013)

——, and Christopher Fee, *The Goddess: Myths of the Great Mother* (London, 2016)

——, and Jake Page, *God: Myths of the Male Divine* (New York and Oxford, 1996)

——, and Jake Page, *Goddess: Myths of the Female Divine* (New York and Oxford, 1994)

——, and Jake Page, *The Mythology of Native North America* (Norman, OK, 1997)

——, ed., *Encyclopedia of Psychology and Religion*, 3 vols (New York, 2014)

Leick, Gwendolyn, *Sex and Eroticism in Mesopotamian Literature* (London and New York, 1994)

Lindow, John, *Norse Mythology: A Guide to the Gods, Heroes, Rituals, and Beliefs* (Oxford and New York, 2001)

Markale, Jean, *The Great Goddess: Reverence of the Divine Feminine from the Paleolithic to the Present* (Rochester, VT, 1999)

Mellaart, James, *Catal Huyuk: A Neolithic Town in Anatolia* (New York, 1967)

Nilsson, Martin, *A History of Greek Religion* (New York, 1965)

——, *The Mycenaean Origins of Greek Mythology* (Berkley, CA, 1972)

Ovid, *Ovid's Metamorphoses*, trans. Charles Boer (Dallas, TX, 1989)

Parrinder, Geoffrey, *African Mythology* (London, 1967)

Pelton, Robert D., *The Trickster in West Africa: A Study in Mythic Irony and Sacred Delight* (Berkeley, CA, 1980)

Pinch, Geraldine, *Egyptian Mythology: A Guide to the Gods, Goddesses, and Traditions of Ancient Egypt* (Oxford and New York, 2002)

Plutarch, *Moralia*, vol. V (Cambridge, MA, 1959)

Popol Vuh: The Sacred Book of the Ancient Quiche Maya (copied from the oral Mayan language in Latin script by Father Francisco Ximenez, from the Spanish translation of Adrian Recinos), trans. Delia Goetz and Sylvanus G. Morley (Norman, OK, 1950)

Puhvel, Jaan, *Comparative Mythology* (Baltimore, MD, 1987)

Radin, Paul, *The Trickster: A Study in American Indian Mythology* (New York, 1988)

Ramanujan, A. K., *The Collected Essays of A. K. Ramanujan*, ed. Vinay Dharwadker (Oxford and New York, 1999)

Read, Kay Almere, and Jason J. Gonzalez, *Mesoamerican Mythology: A Guide to the Gods, Heroes, Rituals, and Beliefs of Mexico and Central America* (New York and Oxford, 2000)

Sanders, N. K., ed. and trans., *The Epic of Gilgamesh* (London, 1972)

Scheub, Harold, *Trickster and Hero: Two Characters in the Oral and Written Traditions of the World* (Madison, WI, 2012)

Shanhaijing (The Classic of Mountains and Seas), trans. Anne Birrell (London, 2000)

Smith, W. Ramsay, *Myths and Legends of the Australian Aborigines* (Mineola, NY, 2003)

Sturluson, Snorri, *The Prose Edda: Tales from Norse Mythology*, trans. Jean I. Young (Berkeley, CA, 1974)

The Táin, trans. Thomas Kinsella (Oxford, 1970)

The Táin, trans. Ciaran Carson (London, 2007)

Virgil, *Aeneid*, trans. Robert Fitzgerald (New York, 1990)

Walker, Barbara G., *The Woman's Encyclopedia of Myths and Secrets* (San Francisco, CA, 1983)

Wasilewska, Ewa, *Creation Stories of the Middle East* (London and Philadelphia, PA, 2000)

Williams, George M., *Handbook of Hindu Mythology* (Oxford and New York, 1993)

Williams, Mark, *Ireland's Immortals: A History of the Gods of Irish Myth* (Princeton, NJ, 2017)

Wolkstein, Diane, and Samuel Noah Kramer, *Inanna, Queen of Heaven and Earth: Her Stories and Hymns from Sumer* (New York, 1983)

Yang, Lihui, and Deming An, with Jessica Anderson Turner, *Chinese Mythology* (Oxford and New York, 2005)

Zaehner, R. C., *Hinduism* (New York and Oxford, 1966)

Zolbrod, Paul, *Dine Bahane: The Navajo Creation Story* (Albuquerque, NM, 1984)

INDEX

Page numbers in *italics* refer to illustrations